The new generational contract

The new generational contract

Intergenerational relations, old age and welfare

Edited by
Alan Walker
University of Sheffield

First published in 1996 by UCL Press

UCL Press Limited
University College London
Gower Street
London WC1E 6BT

and
1900 Frost Road, Suite 101
Bristol
Pennsylvania 19007-1598

The name of University College London (UCL) is a registered
trade mark used by UCL Press with the consent of the owner.

British Library Cataloguing in Publication Data
A catalogue record for this book is available from the British Library.

Library of Congress Cataloging-in-Publication Data are available.

ISBNs:
1-85728-211-6 HB
1-85728-212-4 PB

Typeset in Palatino.
Printed and bound by
Biddles Ltd, Guildford and King's Lynn, England.

To the memory of Maggie Kuhn

Contents

Preface   ix

List of tables   xi

Contributors   xiii

Introduction: the new generational contract   1
Alan Walker

1   Intergenerational relations and the provision of welfare   10
     Alan Walker

2   Intergenerational relationships past and present   37
     Richard Wall

3   Does Britain have a welfare generation?   56
     John Hills

4   Ties that bind   81
     Dorothy Jerrome

5   Obligations and support within families   100
     Hazel Qureshi

6   Inheritance and financial transfer in families   120
     Janet Finch

7   Housing inheritance in Britain: its scale, size, and future   135
     Chris Hamnett

8   Intergenerational relations in the labour market:
     the attitudes of employers and older workers   159
     Philip Taylor and Alan Walker

9 Learning generations: age and education   187
    Tom Schuller

10 Intergenerational conflict and the welfare state: 206
    American and British perspectives
    Chris Phillipson

Bibliography   221
Index   237

Preface

This collection of essays has been put together under the auspices of the Sociology and Social Policy Section of the British Association for the Advancement of Science (BA). Following an appointment as vice president of the Sociology Section in 1988 I proposed the establishment of a separate Social Policy Section. After due deliberation the BA decided to make the Sociology Section a joint one with Social Policy. This seemed entirely appropriate given the heavy reliance of social policy on the core social science discipline of sociology. I was invited to be president in the first year of the newly constituted section.

The main task of the president is to organize a symposium at the annual BA meetings. Thus the main aims in putting together the papers that form the nucleus of this book were to focus on a topic that straddles social analysis and social policy, to help to redress the longstanding neglect in British sociology of studies of ageing and older people, and to begin to fill the remarkable lacuna of sociological and social policy commentary on the profound changes taking place in human relations across the generations. Intergenerational relations between kin and the social contract between age cohorts form essential elements of social cohesion and, therefore, it is amazing that they have been virtually neglected since the early 1960s by social scientists, particularly British ones (with honourable exceptions such as Peter Laslett).

I am very grateful to the original seven speakers for their patience during the process of negotiating a publication contract and to all contributors for revising their papers so carefully. Thanks are also due to the BA recorder, John Cooper, and the then secretary, Andrew Webster, for their support, to Justin Vaughan for his firm but understanding role as publisher (which has been exemplary in every respect), to Marg Walker for extensive technical assistance in preparing the manuscript for publication, and to Christine Firth for her skilled copy-editing. Apologies must be given to Carol, Alison and Christopher for the neglect that this sort of enterprise inevitably entails.

The book is dedicated to the memory of Maggie Kuhn, who died on 22 April 1995. Maggie was the founder and leader of the Gray Panthers in the USA. She was fighting for social justice right up to her death at the age of 89 and provides a continuing inspiration to us all. She called old age a "triumph, not a disease" and although she is best known for her work with the Gray Panthers she did not believe in older people campaigning solely in their own interest. As she put it, "I feel strongly that the old must not simply advocate on their own behalf. We must act as the elders of the tribe, looking out for the best interests of the future and preserving the precious compact between the generations" (Kuhn 1991: 209). She should be remembered as one of this century's great heroes.

Alan Walker
University of Sheffield

List of tables

I.1 Those in employment have a duty to ensure, through   4
    contributions or taxes, that older people have a decent
    standard of living

2.1 Living arrangements of persons aged 65+:   42
    England and Wales, sixteenth to twentieth centuries

2.2 Living arrangements during middle and old age: 48
    English rural populations before 1800

2.3 Living arrangements during middle and old age: 49
    England and Wales 1891

2.4 Living arrangements during middle and old age.   50
    England and Wales 1921

2.5 Living arrangements during middle and old age: 51
    England and Wales 1981

3.1 Age cohorts used in the analysis   61

3.2 Cumulative net receipts by cohort in 1991   68

3.3 Projected total spending on education, health and   70
    social security 1991 to 2041

3.4 Cumulative net receipts by cohort in 2041   71

3.5 Projected life-time receipts and tax payments until 2041   75
    (1991 spending pattern maintained)

LIST OF TABLES

3.6 Projected life-time receipts and tax payments until 2041   77
     (variations to 1991 spending pattern)

5.1 Sources of informal care   105

5.2 Providers of care   106

7.1 Asset composition of estates passing at death, 1988–9   145

7.2 Number and value of estates passing at death   148

7.3 Residential property passing at death, 1987–8   150

7.4 Distribution of housing inheritance by class   151

7.5 Comparisons of different projected levels of housing   152
     inheritance: number of non-spouse transfers

8.1 Labour force participation of older men and women   161
     in Britain, 1951–93

8.2 Respondents by current employment status   164

9.1 Highest qualification by age group   195

9.2 Received job training in previous four weeks   196

9.3 Received job training in previous four weeks   196
     (% of all dependent employees)

Contributors

Janet Finch, Vice Chancellor, University of Keele.

Chris Hammett, Professor of Geography, King's College London.

John Hills, Reader in Economics and Social Policy, London School of Economics.

Dorothy Jerrome, Senior Lecturer in Social Gerontology, University of Southampton.

Chris Phillipson, Professor of Applied Social Studies and Social Gerontology, University of Keele.

Hazel Qureshi, Assistant Director, Social Policy Research Unit, University of York.

Tom Schuller, Professor of Continuing Education, University of Edinburgh.

Philip Taylor, Research Fellow, Policy Studies Institute.

Alan Walker, Professor of Social Policy, University of Sheffield.

Richard Wall, Senior Research Associate, Cambridge Group for the History of Population and Social Structure.

Introduction:
the new generational contract

Alan Walker

In the late twentieth century, old age has again emerged as a lightning rod for the storms of liberal capitalism and middle-class identity. (Cole 1992: 235)

The subject of this book is one that both resonates throughout human history and yet is of immediate concern to politicians and other policy-makers in all western societies: the contract between generations. Relations between generations have been the source of both extraordinary solidarity and major conflict throughout history. The biblical examples of Job and his sceptical sons, the unfortunate Oedipus of Greek legend and King Lear's mistaken confidence in his daughters are longstanding indications of the tenuous nature of some generational relations. Yet the post-war sociological research literature on the family has demonstrated over and over again that intra- and intergenerational relations within the family are, by far, the most important source of care and tending for those in need. This continuity between human societies, East and West, is remarkable and has survived momentous social and economic changes in the twentieth century. This is not to suggest that modern family relationships are characterized by consensus: far from it, feminist sociological analysis has demonstrated the inherent conflict between the sexes on which the caring relationship is founded – an issue that is explored later in this volume.

So, what Mannheim called the "problem of generations" is an age-old one. But, as the twentieth century draws to its conclusion, it appears that industrial societies are confronting a new generational

1

crossroads. While the 1960s witnessed the classic generational conflict between the incumbents of economic security and positions of authority and their successors – the middle aged and youth – in the late 1980s and 1990s attention shifted to the oldest age group. Now the debate about generations is being focused increasingly on the economic, social and moral obligations of the middle aged and young to the increasing numbers of older people and, in turn, the senior citizens' or future senior citizens' obligations to younger people.

The rhetoric of this new confrontation between age groups has already become outspokenly harsh as can be gauged, for example, from media coverage. In 1990 a *Guardian* leader asked "Will the Third World War be a war between generations rather than states?" In the same year *Newsweek* carried a cover story in the USA proclaiming "Greedy Geezers" and in a similar vein Forbes: "Cry, baby: the Greedy Geezers are taking your inheritance". In the previous year *Der Spiegel* had a front page story titled "The struggle of generations: young against old". Although the most colourful rhetoric has been American, the issue of intergenerational equity is relevant to all western societies because of the social contract between generations implicit within the welfare state. This social policy contract is based on intergenerational transfers of resources through the mediums of taxation and social expenditure. Of course the social contract is not like any normal contract in that it is imposed by the state on those in employment rather than being freely negotiated and is heavily sanctioned by the work ethic (or what should more correctly be called the paid employment ethic). Thus there is not a direct exchange between the generations involved, the relationship between them is mediated by the state. Detractors are correct in pointing out that the generational contract lacks explicit content, precision and forms of redress. According to Laslett & Fishkin (1992b: 2) "If a contract is to settle things, people should be able to rely on some account of what to expect and what will be expected of them" (see also Thomson 1992). But, while such legalistic requirements would be in the best interests of all concerned, the absence of such codification does not mean that both institutions and individuals do not behave as if such a contract exists. Thus the welfare state has operated as a system of intergenerational as well as intragenerational transfers and, therefore, has institutionalized and encouraged the expectation of reciprocity.

The essence of the contract was clearly expressed by one of the main architects of the post-war welfare state, William Beveridge (1942: 6):

"Social security must be achieved by cooperation between the State and the individual. The State should offer security in return for service and contribution". It is the widespread acceptance of this dual responsibility and the perceived deservingness of pensioners that gives the social contract its legitimacy in the eyes of tax-payers and voters; it being most improbable that the high level of support the social contract enjoys in the UK and other European countries could be sustained by the rule of law alone. The most recent expression of this was witnessed in the European Union (EU)-wide Eurobarometer surveys of public attitudes to ageing and older people (Walker 1993c). The general public in each member state were asked to what extent they agreed or disagreed with the proposition that those in employment have a duty to ensure, through the contributions or taxes they pay, that older people have a decent standard of living. The results, shown in Table I.1, display a remarkably high level of solidarity in the UK and other EU countries alike and suggest that the social contract is in good shape. There was a slight tendency for those aged 15–24 and 25–34, across the EU as a whole, not to be as strong in their agreement as older age groups. However, these younger age groups were more likely than the older ones to agree slightly, so the overall consensus on the importance of intergenerational solidarity was maintained. Other data from the Eurobarometer surveys show that a majority of the general public in the UK not only support the social contract but also believe that it should be improved. For example, well over half of the public said that pensions are too low and should be raised, even if this means increasing taxes. A similar proportion said that pensions should be close to the average wage for people still in employment (Walker 1993c: 19–20).

This macrosocial policy contract mirrors a micro-level one between kin whereby, for various reasons including reciprocity and affection, adult children provide care for their ageing parents. This intergenerational duty of care may be traced back to the biblical precept to "honour" one's parents and the expectation of filial piety may be found in a wide range of religions and philosophies from Judaism to Confucianism (Cohen 1993). In the 1990s, despite its demonstrably unfair impact on female carers, the intergenerational caring relationship remains the main source of care for older people in western welfare state societies and, in most eastern countries, it is the only form of care available.

There is nothing new about either form of the social contract: one is as ancient as civilization itself while the other has been institutional-

3

Table I.1 Those in employment have a duty to ensure, through contributions or taxes, that older people have a decent standard of living.

	EC12	Belgium	Denmark	France	Germany	Greece	Ireland	Italy	Luxem-bourg	Nether-lands	Portugal	Spain	UK
Agree strongly	37.0	32.5	60.1	25.9	30.4	39.4	40.7	38.4	34.2	42.4	41.2	45.7	45.9
Agree slightly	42.8	42.7	29.8	51.2	48.4	35.0	40.9	40.1	44.8	38.2	32.3	38.1	37.2
Disagree slightly	9.0	13.8	6.3	13.0	11.4	8.3	5.8	6.9	10.6	9.8	10.0	4.4	6.2
Disagree strongly	8.6	4.1	2.0	4.6	3.6	4.2	1.7	2.7	3.4	4.0	7.8	2.8	3.1
Don't know	7.6	6.9	1.8	5.3	6.2	13.1	10.9	11.1	7.0	5.6	8.7	9.1	7.5

Source: Walker 1993c: 15

ized by the introduction of welfare regimes of various types (though some early forms of welfare provision, such as the English Poor Law, sometimes included a formal requirement that adult children should accept financial responsibility for their aged parents). Nor is there anything new about macro-age group or cohort conflicts which are recorded, in the UK, 400 years ago (Thomas 1976). More recently, in 1956, the United Nations (UN) expressed concern about the "psychological effects" on those in employment of the increase in pensions contributions necessary in an ageing society. However, the combination of increased life expectancy, decline in fertility and political concerns among policy-makers about the fiscal consequences of population ageing is unique to the late twentieth century. This has profound implications for both caring relationships within families, which are being extended, and the provision of public pensions, health and social care. It is resulting in revisions being made to the social contract implicit within different welfare regimes and increased expectations being placed on both intra- and intergenerational carers within the family. Thus the microsocial contract is being altered as a result of changes in public policy and this has major implications for the micro-level contract. In some countries the shape of the new generational contract is becoming clear already. For example in the UK it is being made obvious to those currently of working age that they cannot rely on the social contract to ensure economic security when they retire:

> In the West, governments play a key role in the provision of pensions. Ageing populations create pressure for higher expenditure on pensions, leading to higher taxes falling on fewer workers. And yet, in a world of global markets and capital flows, governments cannot increase taxes significantly without damaging national competitiveness. In these circumstances, individuals will not be able to look to the state to fund improvements in their living standards in old age. (Department of Trade and Industry 1995: para 6.2)

As a result of population ageing, changes in the provision of health and social care services and changes in the politics of gender, particularly with regard to the labour market, the caring relationship within families is also in transition. In fact it looks as if the intention of some governments to create a new generational contract is on collision

5

course with the changes underway in generational patterns within families.

The key purpose of this volume is to subject the generational contract, and particularly the changes currently being made to it, to sustained analysis. The two dimensions of intergenerational relations and welfare and the interconnections between them are analyzed from the perspectives of history, sociology, economics, anthropology, education and policy analysis. Thereby it is intended to provide the reader with a multidimensional picture of the connections between intergenerational relations and, broadly defined, welfare.

Before introducing the plan of the book it is necessary to make a distinction between generations and cohorts. So far I have been using the term "generations" in its lay generic sense – to indicate groups of different ages in society. But to understand recent developments in the generational contract it is important to be more precise conceptually. Thus we may use the term "cohort" to refer to those individuals who have been born at roughly the same point in chronological time, while the term "generation" denotes the single step in ranked-descent ordering of individuals within families; or put more simply, "generation" reflects microsocial roles and interactions between age groups within families (Bengston et al. 1985, Daniels 1988).

Although this volume focuses primarily on the concepts of cohort and generation, in order to redress their neglect in the sociological and social policy literature, we are not proposing that they have any special analytical power. Birth cohort or generation may exert important influences on the way individuals understand and interpret everyday life (Becker 1987) but, of course, there are other powerful frames of reference as well. Thus it is important to caution against cohort-determinism in which it is assumed that members of the same age cohort experience age in exactly the same way. An interest in age group stratification should not blind us to variations within cohorts. This caution derives from the political economy of ageing thesis (Guillemard 1980, Walker 1981, Estes et al. 1982, Phillipson 1982, Myles 1984, Dannefer 1988) which arose in part as a critique of the analytical limitations of age stratification theory. Notwithstanding the important intellectual contribution made by age stratification theory, its excessively narrow concentration on chronological age and birth year divert attention from both individual responses to the ageing process and differences within age cohorts deriving from macrostructural factors such as social class, sex, gender and race. Thus in

6

focusing on the importance of relations between generations we must not fall into a "cohort trap" by assuming either that relations between members of successive birth cohorts are characteristic of all such intergenerational relations involving those cohorts, or that membership of a particular cohort is necessarily more influential than other factors in determining the nature of these relations (Riley & Riley 1993).

Having cautioned against over-emphasizing the importance of generations it is remarkable that, relatively speaking, this topic has been given so little attention in the post-war sociology and social policy literature. Indeed, until 1991, the analysis of intergenerational relations had not progressed far beyond the pioneering work of Shanas and her colleagues (Shanas & Streib 1965, Shanas et al. 1968). This neglect was particularly the case with regard to macro-level age cohort relations. But, as Kohli (1993) has pointed out, population ageing makes the issue of solidarity between generations even more salient and, in the wake of the rhetorical attack on the generational contract in the US, has come a series of scientific analyses that have contributed substantially to public knowledge on this subject (see for example Bengston & Achenbaum 1993, Cohen 1993, Marmor et al. 1994). The importance of the issue has been recognized by international economic agencies such as the Organization for Economic Cooperation and Development (OECD 1994) and World Bank (1994) and, at a supra-national level, by the Commission of the European Communities (1990: 4):

> Ageing will affect two critical components of the economy: the labour market and public social welfare expenditure. A substantial degree of solidarity between generations and social integration is needed to cope with problems in these two fields.

Plan of volume

The authors in this volume address both the macro and micro features of intergenerational relations and welfare. The main elements of the new generational contract that is emerging in the late twentieth century are examined in separate chapters – the social (welfare state) contract, employment and the changing life-course, education, family relationships, the provision of informal care, and support and inheritance. Chapter 1 operates as an extended introduction to the twin dimensions of generational relations and their interaction in determining welfare. It is argued that social policy and state ideology in particular plays a key role in the social construction of both intergenerational conflict at the macro-level and the caring relationship within families. At the same time this chapter attempts to transcend the macro–micro distinction by pointing to the interaction of agency and structure in determining the nature of the social contract between generations. Richard Wall's historical perspective (Ch. 2) provides an antidote to the "world we have lost syndrome" that permeates much contemporary discussion of generational relations. He shows, among other things, the historical continuity between past and present in the provision of social and financial support by a small select group of relatives. John Hills' economic analysis (Ch. 3) challenges the central premises of the "welfare generation" thesis and the generational equity debate: that the baby boom generation has either "captured" the welfare state (Thomson 1991, 1992) or is "born to pay" for it (Longman 1987). On the contrary he shows that the welfare state in Britain has been remarkably even-handed between the generations. Hills also shows the dramatic impact of government policies aimed at reducing the size of the welfare state on the levels of support that future generations may look forward to under the social contract.

Chapters 4 and 5 focus on intergenerational relations between kin. Dorothy Jerrome, drawing on the British Mass Observation Archive, illustrates the growth of diversity in family life and relationships and calls for a more flexible concept of the family. Hazel Qureshi examines obligations and support within families. She argues on the basis of historical and contemporary research that attempts to impose a duty of care on families, which run counter to prevailing beliefs about what should reasonably be expected, are bound to fail. Her analysis exposes the need for more pro-active health and social services and the need to provide support in a preventive form as well as a reactive one.

Chapters 6 and 7 examine the neglected but, in practice, sometimes vexed issue of inheritance. Janet Finch uses her pioneering work on inheritance, property and family relationships to show that, in "ordinary" families, inheritance is both too diffuse and comes too late to have a marked impact on life chances. Chris Hamnett focuses on housing and, using Inland Revenue data, shows that predictions of a massive increase in housing inheritance are false and one of the main reasons is the sale of houses to pay for care.

Chapter 8 takes a preliminary look at intergenerational relations in the labour market. This issue will grow in importance as the workforce ages and, as Phillip Taylor and I argue, employers will have to alter their youth bias to reflect this change. Tom Schuller (Ch. 9) provides a critique of the preparatory conception of education, which links it closely to youth, which dominates both expert and lay educational thinking. He puts a powerful case for the notion of an intergenerational educational contract and suggests practical measures to achieve it.

Finally Chris Phillipson critically analyzes the intergenerational conflict thesis from US and British perspectives. His Chapter 10 rounds off the volume by arguing for a period of renewal in terms of generational politics. In order to commence this process it is necessary to recognize that a different type of life-course is under construction, one in which the labels of "worker" and "pensioner" become even more problematic than at present. As Phillipson argues, responsibility for population ageing should not be offloaded on to particular generations or age cohorts: "Ageing is an issue for generations, but it is also a question to be solved with generations."

CHAPTER 1

Intergenerational relations and the provision of welfare

Alan Walker

Introduction

This chapter focuses on the social "intergenerational" contract that lies at the heart of all western welfare state regimes and the changes it is undergoing currently. The two sections of the chapter reflect the conceptual distinction between macro-age cohorts and microsocial roles within families outlined in the introduction. In the first section it is argued that while the classic "problem of generations" (Bengston 1993) is concerned with relations within families, the late twentieth century is witnessing the emergence of a wholly new problem between age cohorts and the main battleground is the distributory mechanisms of the traditional welfare state. A new contract is being forged between the age cohorts of workers and pensioners. Secondly, this new contract between age cohorts and the restructuring of welfare systems that lies behind it have profound implications for generational relations within families, especially when coupled, as they are, with the dramatic increases in life expectancy during the twentieth century. Thus it is argued that the new contract between age cohorts is at odds with the changes taking place in generational relations within families.

There is universal agreement that the unique late-twentieth-century phenomenon of population ageing has raised questions about the main element of this contract: public pension provision and, to a lesser extent, the provision of health and social care. However, the precise nature and outcome of the challenge facing the social contract is subject to a wide variety of interpretations; ranging from those who argue, apocalyptically, that the demise of the welfare state is nigh (Thomson 1989), to those who regard the notion of "intergenerational equity" as, at best, based on the shakiest of empirical and theoretical grounds and, at worst, representing a dangerous diversion of policy-makers' and the public's attention from the major sources of inequality and dependent economic and social status (Achenbaum 1989, Quadagno 1989, Walker 1990a). What is beyond question is that the social contract is currently the subject of "renegotiation" and modification in the majority of western societies, though the extent of the changes introduced or planned differs substantially between countries, even within the European Union (Walker 1990b).

Throughout much of the sociological literature on what is now widely accepted as the "new problem of generations" there is a relatively uncritical acceptance of both the hypothesis of conflict between age cohorts in the distribution of public resources and the link between demographics and policy change in the realm of welfare. Hence a key aim of this chapter is to question the motivation behind the revisions to the public pensions contract. It is suggested that, at least as far as Britain and other EU countries are concerned, these changes have little or nothing to do with "intergenerational" conflict. This leads on to a contrast between the public debate concerning "intergenerational equity" in the USA and EU countries where it has hardly surfaced.

It is argued that the primary concern of policy-makers is with the perceived burden of pensions on public expenditure rather than any manifest concern about distributional justice between age cohorts. Thus, for largely ideological reasons, an economic-demographic imperative has been manufactured in some countries, with the aid of international economic agencies, to facilitate the restructuring of their welfare states. In the name of this imperative some countries have set about rewriting the post-war social contract between age cohorts. Rather than being "rooted in life-course processes" (Bengston et al. 1991: 255) the "intergenerational equity" debate should be regarded as a socio-political construct. Seen in this light it is not surprising that, during the 1980s, the USA led the way in discussions of "intergenerational equity". Concerns such as these sit more comfortably within the context of an individualistic welfare tradition and pluralistic political system, particularly one under neo-liberal leadership, than they do within the more solidaristic or collectivist welfare traditions and corporatist political systems of northern Europe. Britain in

11

the 1980s and early 1990s represented a peculiar hybrid case: a traditional solidaristic welfare state under neo-liberal management and, therefore, welfare restructuring took an extreme form with the aim being to make the British welfare state more like the "market-orientated states" of Australia, Canada and the USA (Therborn & Roebroek 1986, Walker 1990c). Therefore it is argued here that whether the social contract survives or is repudiated in different societies is largely a matter of social and economic policy.

The second section of this chapter focuses on the micro-sociological dimension of generational relations, though one of my main intentions is to emphasize the interconnection between agency and social structure. As far as intergenerational relations within families are concerned it is commonly assumed that the informal contract between generations is determined primarily by the norms of reciprocity and affection: because my parents cared for me as a child I must care for them in their advanced old age (Bengston et al. 1991). However, research may be used to demonstrate that, while affection and reciprocity are critical determinants of the *quality* of intergenerational relations within the family, the *provision* of care by female kin cannot be explained without reference to macro-structural determinants. In other words interpersonal caring relationships within the family are as much an arena for state intervention as financial transfers between age cohorts, though of course the forms that these interventions take are very different.

The "natural" reciprocity and altruism of female kin has figured centrally, as a social construction, in both the history of the welfare state and in recent attempts to restructure it and enlarge the role of the informal sector in caring for older people (Land & Rose 1985, Walker 1987, Langan & Ostner 1991, Lewis 1993). However, faced with the momentous changes underway in family structure, as a result of population ageing and other socio-economic changes, this simple social construction will be harder and harder to reproduce and sustain, not least because the process of restructuring welfare provision itself is imposing additional strains on the caring relationship between them. For example the National Health Service (NHS) has been criticized for abandoning long-term geriatric care in order to reduce costs, with the inevitable result that families either have to shoulder the physical burden of care or have to contribute financially to their relatives' private care (Henwood 1992, Walker 1995). Since, like the macrosocial contract between age cohorts, interpersonal caring contracts between family members are not negotiated in a political, economic and ideological vacuum, whether or not this generational contract remains intact over the coming decades is largely a matter of social and economic policy.

The social contract, the welfare state and demographic change

Most welfare states originated in pension provision for older people and in all OECD countries in the 1990s, this group is the main beneficiary of social expenditure. In fact, in European welfare states, the social contract is primarily a public pensions contract between age cohorts. (In the USA the absence of a national health insurance or care programme ensures that the cost of health care provision to older people remains central to the debate about the social contract.) Thus, for the purposes of this account, the "social contract" is interpreted as being a social policy contract based on intercohort transfers of resources through the mediums of taxation and social expenditure. In other words the social contract is only one, reified, form of contract between generations. Moreover, as explained in more detail later, social norms concerning the role of the family in the care of older relatives as well as children, which are reinforced by state policy, have the effect of supporting the individual-level contract between generations while, at the same time, limiting the scope of the macrosocial policy contract.

Although public transfers are only one of the four "pillars" on which retirement income is founded (Reday-Mulvey 1990) they are the largest one in the majority of OECD countries. The proportion of the gross income of retired households deriving from social security (insurance and social assistance) ranges from over 80 per cent in Sweden and Germany, to 68 per cent in the UK, to around 50 per cent in Canada and the USA (OECD 1988a: 55). Of course the social contract on which these transfers are based is not like any normal contract in that it is imposed by the state on those in employment rather than being freely negotiated and is heavily sanctioned by the work ethic, or what should more correctly be called the paid employment ethic. (Thus there is not a direct exchange between the cohorts involved; the relationship between them is mediated by the state.) The essence of the contract was clearly expressed by one of the main architects of the post-war welfare state, Beveridge (1942: 6), as was quoted on page 3.

When the first pension schemes were introduced in the late nineteenth century they benefited only those who had the good fortune to survive beyond average life expectancy. The twentieth century has seen not only growth in the numbers of older people in the population of western societies but also a rising proportion of those eligible for pensions being able to collect them and then subsequently to go on doing so for longer periods (though there remain significant differences in mortality rates between social classes). The issue of the future of the public pensions contract between age cohorts has become particularly salient in the late twentieth century because of the combination of three trends. First, there is the dramatic increase in life expectancy in western societies. This means that there are many more older people living to advanced old age. In the UK between 1951 and 1991 the numbers aged 65 and over increased by 66 per cent while those aged 85 and over increased by 300 per cent. The projected increases from 1991 to 2021 are 19 per cent and 50 per cent respectively. This ageing of the older population is resulting in a functional separation of age cohorts in retirement, with those over 85 being more likely than younger groups to suffer from disablement (33 per cent are unable to go outdoors compared with 8 per cent of the whole 65 plus group), poverty and isolation. Secondly, there is the decline in fertility, which means that there are fewer young labour market entrants and fewer workers per pensioner than in previous decades (also, within families, there are fewer second and third generation family members to care for older relatives in need). Thirdly, partly as a result of these factors, there have been increased concerns among policy-makers in all western societies about the fiscal consequences of population ageing. In some countries this has been popularized in terms of the distribution of welfare state resources between cohorts or "generational equity". In other words the issue of distributional equity between age cohorts is "new" to western societies because of the combination in the late twentieth century of these three factors. Age cohort conflicts are certainly not new in historical terms (see below p. 29 and Ch. 2).

Even in the absence of generational equity rhetoric, population ageing has been greeted with pessimism and alarm in many western societies; this has prompted action among a broad range of western countries to modify their public pension schemes and, thereby, the social contract on which these schemes are based. Examples of the more pessimistic response to the socio-economic implications of societal ageing include the OECD (1988a; see also OECD 1994, World Bank 1994):

14

Under existing regulations the evolution of public pension schemes is likely to put a heavy and increasing burden on the working population in coming decades. Such a financial strain may put intergenerational solidarity – a concept on which all public retirement provisions are based – at risk. (OECD 1988a: 102)

While the following is typical of the more apocalyptic version of this theme:

If no action is taken to deal with the incipient crisis of population ageing, then it seems certain that western societies will experience major social and economic dislocation, and they may experience this relatively soon. (Johnson et al. 1989: 13)

In the light of such dire predictions the actions taken so far by western nations, with one or two notable exceptions, look remarkably modest. For example several EU countries, including Denmark and Germany, have increased their retirement ages or are in the process of doing so. Others, such as France and Italy, are contemplating such a change. Action has been taken or is planned in France and Spain to make the qualification conditions for pensions more stringent; while some other countries, including Belgium and the Netherlands, have restricted the level of pensions available (Walker 1990b). This brief review of recent policy changes among EU countries draws on more detailed research that demonstrates that just as there are "multiple paths to higher pen sion spending" (Pampel et al. 1990: 547) then the reverse is also true.

The new social contract and welfare state restructuring[1]

Despite encouragement from international economic agencies such as the International Monetary Fund (IMF) and OECD and high profile political rhetoric in some countries, especially the USA, concerning "intergenerational equity", the extent of the modifications to the social contract are relatively minor in the majority of western countries. So far at least the new social contract between age cohorts is not very different from the old one. There are exceptions though and it is when we distinguish those countries that have led the field in revising the social contract, sometimes in combination with "intergenerational equity" rhetoric, that the connection between the creation of a new social contract between age cohorts and the wider policy of welfare state restructuring can be demonstrated. Stripped of all its euphemisms the newly emerging contract between age cohorts in some western countries consists of cuts in social security for both current and future pensioners and reductions in rights of access to health care.

It was not mere coincidence that the countries that moved furthest and fastest in the 1980s to alter the terms of the social contract were those under neo-liberal economic management – be it Reaganomics in the USA, Thatcherism in Britain or Rogernomics in New Zealand. To a student of social policy the "market-orientated" welfare states, such as Australia, Canada and the USA, are less interesting in their responses to population ageing than those of the collectivist welfare states of northern Europe, simply because the former policies are more predictable. Among the latter Britain stands out as an extreme case. Although the British welfare state (along with those of France, Germany and Italy) has been accurately described as one of "socio-economic mediocrity" in terms of its commitment to the core welfare aims of social security and full employment (Therborn & Roebroek 1986), over the post-war period the state has played a leading role in both the financing and delivery of welfare benefits and services, as in other northern European countries. There is a sharp contrast between the USA and northern European welfare state regimes, which can be gauged not only by well-known differences in institutions and levels of expenditure on the public and private sectors but also from the effectiveness of their public welfare systems. For example the effect of social security spending in the USA is to reduce the proportion of households living below the poverty line by only 10 per cent whereas, in the majority of EU states, social security achieves a reduction in poverty of around 30 per cent (Commission of European Communities 1994). There are also differences in public attitudes to welfare: while Americans and Britons have similar attitudes towards certain aspects of society and the role of government, such as police power, parental rights and free speech, when it comes to the role of the state in welfare the latter are on average twice as likely as the former to favour state intervention and to endorse redistribution (Davies 1986).

It is within this solidaristic context that the Thatcher government, first elected in 1979, set about the restructuring of the British welfare state. Because older people are the main beneficiaries of the largest item of social spending – social security – they quickly became one of the main targets. In 1980 the government changed the method of calculating annual increases in flat-rate national insurance pension from an earnings linked to a prices linked system. In 1988 social assistance payments to older people were reduced and, most importantly, the State Earnings-Related Pension Scheme (SERPS), which was due to reach full maturity in 1998, was severely curtailed. At the same time an "incentive" of 2 per cent of earnings, together with a national insurance contribution rebate of 5.8 per cent, was paid (until 1993) to employees who contract out of SERPS and into a personal (private) pension scheme (Walker 1992, 1993a). As a result some 4 million employees have opted out of SERPS – eight times the government's original estimate. These changes, coupled with a lower growth in the retired population than in most other European countries, have restricted the growth in the projected share of public pension expenditure in national income over the next 50 years to the second lowest in the OECD: from 7.7 per cent in 1984, to 7.6 per cent in 2010 and 11.2 per cent in 2040. Equivalent statistics for the USA are 8.1 per cent, 8.5 per cent and 14.6 per cent; and for Germany 13.7 per cent, 19.7 per cent and 31.1 per cent (OECD 1988a: 35). The cuts in SERPS that will follow the passing of the Pensions Bill 1995 will further reduce the proportion of UK national income being devoted to public pensions.

The restructuring of pension provision in Britain cannot be attributed to the need to curb the generosity of payments to pensioners. In comparison with other EU countries British pensioners fare poorly. For example public pension net replacement rates (pensions as a proportion of earnings in the year before retirement for men with average gross salaries) vary from 92 per cent in Italy, 88 per cent in Belgium, 69 per cent in Germany, to 64 per cent in the UK (joint bottom with Ireland: Walker et al. 1993: 15). It is not surprising, therefore, that poverty remains a major characteristic of old age in Britain, with just over one-half of older people living in or on the margins of poverty (as defined by social assistance levels).

Nor can the restructuring of pensions in Britain be attributed to any overt concern about justice between age cohorts. The issue of "intergenerational equity" did surface in the mid-1980s but only very briefly and in far less sensational terms than in the USA. When the British government reviewed the social security system in 1985, as a prelude to the major restructuring carried through in 1988, it legitimized its proposals for cutting the SERPS with reference to the age cohort contract:

17

Our belief in One Nation means recognizing our responsibilities to *all* the generations represented within it . . . . It would be an abdication of responsibility to hand down obligations to our children which we believe they cannot fulfil. (DHSS 1985a: 18)

There were further fleeting appearances of "intergenerational equity" rhetoric but it has not achieved the same high profile as it did in the USA. It is not unreasonable to expect neo-liberal inspired governments to be rather wary of any concept that invokes the principle of equity. But, in addition, there is no empirical evidence in Britain of any net transfer of state spending from younger to older people. There is no basis for the contention, dramatically expressed by Thomson (1989: 36) that the "welfare generation" has "captured" the welfare state and steered it from being a youth orientated state to one directed towards older people (see also Thomson 1991, 1992). The British welfare state has been neutral, distributionally speaking, between children and older people since the mid-1970s (Johnson & Falkingham 1988a). Any changes in the age cohort distribution of welfare state spending are a reflection of underlying movements in demographic structure rather than being the result of a take-over by "greedy elders" (see Ch. 3).

As far as future social expenditure is concerned a similar picture emerges in all OECD countries. Taking the period 1980–2040, there is no country in which the growth of social expenditure is projected to exceed the rise in the population aged 65 and over (OECD 1988b: 36). For instance, in the USA total social expenditure is projected to rise in real terms by 65 per cent compared with an increase in the older population of 138 per cent. In Germany total spending is set to fall by 3 per cent yet the population aged 65 and over will rise by 31 per cent. Thus, despite the numerous deficiencies in projections, such as these, of the impact of demographic factors on the welfare state – especially the assumptions of constant participation and productivity rates (Binney & Estes 1988, Walker 1990a) – they do not indicate expenditure growth that is out of line with demographic change. In some cases, notably Australia, Canada, Japan and the USA, projected social spending lags considerably behind growth in the older population. This is not surprising since, in retrospect, it was conscious policy decisions concerning eligibility for and levels of benefit that were the major contributors to the increasing share of GDP taken by pensions in the period 1960–85 in all OECD countries; with the demographic factor playing a relatively minor role (Myles 1983, Walker 1990a). In fact it may be argued that older people are entitled to *increased* benefits in line with rising productivity and rises in real incomes among workers, and not just to have their incomes raised in line with inflation (Rosow 1962).

Social construction of an economic-demographic imperative

So, why did the British government impose a new social contract on older people – much diluted from the perspective of current and future pensioners – when there was no public pressure to do so and when, moreover, it was advised to delay doing so by official agencies, the private pension industry and the OECD? The answer is in two parts, the first part of which explains the prevalence of pessimistic attitudes towards population ageing among a wide cross section of western societies and the concomitant growth of ageism. The second part indicates why some governments have gone much further than others in restructuring welfare ostensibly in response to demographic change.

In the first place there is the longstanding economic pessimism concerning public expenditure on the welfare state. This is a phenomenon common to all western societies, to a greater or lesser extent, and for the reasons already outlined has come to be directed more and more at older people as the numbers of them receiving pensions and health care have increased. This seemingly innate pessimism derives from the "public burden" model of welfare that lies at the heart of neo-classical economic assumptions concerning the respective economic contributions of the public and private sectors, and particularly the contention that the former is an unproductive burden on the latter. The official and popular concept of old age stemming from such theories is one of homogeneity, economic dependence and unproductiveness. Thus older people are marginalized economically in the same way that women not in paid employment are, even though both may be performing vital roles in the informal economy. The "first pillar" pensions they receive from the state are regarded economically as a burden, as are the pensioners receiving them, whereas "second pillar" private pensions are not, even though the latter may be heavily subsidized by the state.

The public burden conception of old age in orthodox economics is attributable, in part, to the subordination of social policy to economic policy and the pre-eminence accorded to the latter in the political sphere. Another contributory factor has been individualistic functional theories, such as some variants of the life-cycle approach, whereby economic ability and status are related to specific stages of the life-cycle (Clark & Spengler 1980: 67). It is from this simplistic theory that the demographic imperative originates. Unfortunately the theory has not been amenable to empirical evidence, at least in its unsophisticated form. Most importantly it overlooks the socially constructed relationship between the life-cycle and the labour market and the flexible way in which the definition of productive capacity alters in response to changes in labour supply and particularly the supply of younger workers (Graebner 1980, Phillipson 1982).

Secondly, in some countries ideological change has seriously undermined even the limited "handmaiden" role assigned to the welfare state by Keynesian economics. Neo-monetarism, with its in-built opposition to public expenditure on welfare and supply-side view of the costs of employers' social security contributions, is more important, in countries such as Australia, Britain, Canada and New Zealand, than demography in explaining recent policies aimed at installing a new social contract. The rate of gross domestic product (GDP) growth per annum in Britain required to finance projected increases in social expenditure due to demographic factors is only 0.16 per cent, for the USA it is 0.84 per cent. Even in Canada, which has one of the highest projected social expenditure growths among OECD countries the average annual GDP growth rate required to maintain a constant social expenditure share in the face of demographic change over the next 50 years is only 1.05 per cent (OECD 1988b: 39). Thus, rather than the main pressure deriving from demographic change, it is ideological shifts, particularly in economic orthodoxy, which have altered assumptions about the role of the state with regard to welfare and encouraged some countries to take what looks like, at best, premature action on the social contract. Britain provides a clear example of this triumph of ideology over demography in the restructuring of its pension provision to reduce the role of public pensions and increase that of publicly subsidized private pensions (for a fuller account see Walker 1990a).

The conjunction of these two factors in several western countries since the mid-1980s suggests that concern about population ageing has been artificially amplified as an economic-demographic imperative intended primarily to legitimize policies aimed at creating a new social contract between age cohorts and, more generally, restructuring the welfare state. The dual social functions performed by this amplification process are, on the one hand, to encourage gratitude and political acquiescence on the part of older people and, on the other, to prompt younger adults to provide for their old age in the private market. In addition it diverts attention from the real *ideological* imperative behind policy. Although the British government did dabble briefly with "intergenerational equity" rhetoric it was also explicit about the main reason for its restructuring of pension provision in the 1980s:

> The purpose of these proposals is to achieve a steady transition from the present dependence on state provision to a position in which we as individuals are contributing directly to our own additional pensions and in which we can exercise greater choice in the sort of pension provision we make. (DHSS 1985b: 6)

In other words the main driving force behind the manufacture of a new pensions contract in Britain was the Thatcher government's ideological distaste for public welfare. Further, more recent, support for this conclusion comes from the 1995 Trade and Industry White Paper quoted on p. 5. The converse German case, outlined below, also emphasizes the central place of political ideology in shaping the new contract between age cohorts.

An explanation as to why the Thatcher government was able, with impunity, to carry out a succession of changes to the British pension system throughout the 1980s whereas, in contrast in the USA, the Reagan administration was faced with stiff opposition, requires a detailed analysis of the politics of ageing in Britain (Walker 1992). Briefly there was the ideological determination of the Thatcher government and the social division of pension recipients into different consumption classes, based mainly on previous employment status and income level, which has militated against the development of a unified age-interest lobby. Thus, under the single tier public pension system that prevailed in Britain for most of the post-war period, the interests of working class public pensioners and middle class occupational pensioners were quite different. The maturation of the SERP Scheme would have incorporated the middle class into state pensions but the Thatcher government severely curtailed the scope of that scheme as well as limiting the basic pension. Thus the British public pension system was both vulnerable to cuts by a determined government and less likely than in the USA to be defended by a powerful pensioners' movement.

This ideological and political context is sometimes missing from accounts of macrosocial relations between age cohorts and policy responses to demographic change, yet it is essential if we are to understand the similarities and differences between societies in their responses to demographic change as well as the specific policies adopted by governments, whether in the orthodox economic mould of western capitalism or the more extreme neo-liberal variant. Furthermore policies intended to create a new social contract must be analyzed as one element of the much broader endeavour on the part of some governments to restructure their welfare provision, otherwise they may be wrongly interpreted as simply age discriminatory attacks on the welfare of older people. Although the public burden thesis and "intergenerational equity" rhetoric may encourage ageist attitudes, the impact of current welfare state restructuring on older people is mainly attributable to the fact that they are unfortunate enough to be the main users of the social security and health care systems. Ageist attitudes, however, may be used to legitimate particular outcomes of welfare distribution or restructuring as, for example, when it is claimed that older people have lower income needs compared to younger adults.

"Intergenerational equity"

Some form of welfare state restructuring has taken place in most western societies but, of course, it has been pursued with greatest vigour in those countries under neo-liberal inspired economic management. The mobilization of free-market ideas and policies in Australia, Britain, Canada, New Zealand and the USA during the 1980s produced the main representatives of the genre but many other countries have followed, more selectively, in their wake. The USA is conspicuous because it alone combined neo-liberal economic management with an outspoken debate about "intergenerational equity". This debate has been orchestrated by the pressure group Americans for Generational Equity (AGE) who contend that the flow of federal resources to the oldest age group is increasing every year while the proportion going to children has decreased. Thus to continue spending as much on the elderly is inequitable and will result in intergenerational conflict. In the words of former Colorado Governor Richard Lamm, "We have turned the Biblical account of the prodigal son on its head. We are now faced with the prodigal father".

Why the USA should be the only major western nation so far to have spawned a high profile political lobby group on "intergenerational equity" is a fascinating question; but the answer is likely to reveal more about the political economy of the USA than about relations between North American age cohorts. Research by Pampel and his colleagues (1990) suggests that pluralistic political systems are more amenable to the influence of age structure in determining the level of pension spending than are corporatist systems. Therefore we might expect the US political system, in conjunction with its individualistic welfare tradition, to provide a more conducive setting for an "intergenerational equity" debate than the solidaristic and corporatist approaches characteristic of northern Europe. This conclusion is supported by Marshall et al. (1993) who contrast the emergence of an outspoken lobby on intergenerational equity in the USA with the virtual silence on this issue in Canada. In addition to differences in the political systems of the two countries they point to the greater use in Canada of universal welfare programmes, especially health care, and also the complicity of the US academic community in the promulgation of the intergenerational equity thesis (also see Ch. 10).

Leaving aside the hybrid case of Britain, of all the nations in the European collectivist welfare mould the one that might be regarded as the most likely to repeat the US experience is Germany. It has had the lowest fertility rate among OECD countries since the early 1970s and has the highest projected dependency ratio. Germany spends one of the highest proportions of GDP on pensions in the OECD and is among the countries with the highest proportion of older people in their populations. In addition it has a relatively low labour-force participation rate. Despite these obvious pressures resulting in one or two headlines such as that from *Der Spiegel* quoted earlier, there has been no "intergenerational equity" debate to speak of and certainly nothing to compare with that in the USA (Hinrichs 1991). The main explanatory factors appear to be the solidaristic consensus on the current German welfare system and the absence of an electoral system that would enable a radical neo-liberal government to achieve power.

The concept of "intergenerational equity" has been subjected to sustained criticism (Minkler 1986, Achenbaum 1989, Quadagno 1989, Walker 1990a, Phillipson, Ch. 10 in this volume) and pronounced unsuitable as a basis for either conceptualizing the relationship between age cohorts or for policy development. Moreover in the USA, where it has achieved widest currency, it has signally failed in its main aim to undermine public support for social security (Quadagno 1989:

371, Lomax Cook 1990). This attempt, spearheaded by AGE in the USA, to establish an overtly conflictual relationship between younger and older people and the rather half-hearted stab at doing something similar in Britain, may be regarded as reflections of the same combination of factors that created the much more influential economic-demographic imperative. Thus it is not concern about justice between age cohorts that motivates "intergenerational equity" protagonists but the fiscal implications of ageing: the so-called "burden" of economic dependency in the form of pension costs and the "burden" of physical dependency in the form of health and social care costs. In short population ageing is regarded as a threat to accumulation. Marmor and his colleagues (1994) have shown that intergenerational equity rhetoric is a product of the politics of social security retrenchment. As AGE president James Jones (1988: 7) himself has made clear, it is the stagnation of production and low investment in the USA that are the main causes of his group's gloomy prognoses for North American society.

Such concerns are not new ones, nor is the tendency in times of recession to regard older people as a burden (see Chs 2 and 10). In Britain there is evidence from the sixteenth century that when village communities were faced with economic hardship older people were sometimes marginalized and their financial relief portrayed as a "burden on the community" (Thomas 1976). The social construction of age cohort conflicts predates Americans for Generational Equity by at least 400 years and is not a phenomenon associated uniquely with late-twentieth-century population ageing. In the mid-1950s the United Nations (1956) expressed concern about the "psychological effects" on those in employment of the increase in pensions contributions necessary in an ageing society. Of course it is precisely these considerations that lay behind the main tool of demographers and economists in this field – the deeply flawed dependency ratio – and the scientific, governmental and popular construction of older people as a burden on middle-age cohorts is perpetuated by its use.

The "intergenerational equity" thesis derives from the predominantly economic concerns of the public burden model of welfare. It is merely a politically expedient use of demographic change to conceal, on the one hand, the falling welfare surplus and, on the other, welfare restructuring. Additional support for this conclusion comes from the lacuna of policies accompanying "intergenerational equity" rhetoric that would improve the material position of the younger age groups that are said to be the target of the campaign (Quadagno 1989).

24

Policies aimed at redistributing resources according to goals such as social justice, or "interclass equity", are simply not on the agenda of those countries in the process of restructuring their welfare states. Thus older people are being caricatured as "greedy elders" and used, to some extent, as scapegoats for both economic failure and ideological opposition to social policies that would meet the needs of older and younger people alike (Binstock 1983). This hostile policy climate has led to the reversal of compassionate stereotypes of older people to their portrayal, instead, as a powerful and greedy generation (Binstock 1994).

Intergenerational relations and the provision of care

Having analyzed the motivations behind the development of a new social contract between age cohorts attention shifts now to the second dimension of generational relations· relationships between kin. The centre of focus here is the caring relationship within the family. However, although these two dimensions of generational relations have been delineated, one of the primary functions of this chapter is to argue against their common separation in the literature. While there are distinct macro- and microsocial features of generational relations one effect of this dichotomous scientific construction of the social world is to underplay the degree of interaction between them. As with the newly emerging pensions contract in western societies the role of ideology is central to the social reproduction of the caring relationship.[2] In this sphere, however, the state has been much more cautious about overt intervention in what is portrayed as an essentially private domain. Thus the lack in most western countries of macro-level policies that successfully share care between the family and the state reflects the latter's objective to minimize its financial commitment in the field of social care and to sustain the primacy of the family. The continued absence of such policies means that unnecessary strains are placed on the caring relationships between kin as they respond to the fundamental changes in intergenerational patterns and responsibilities being brought about by socio-demographic change.

Reciprocity and affect in generational relations

It is widely accepted in the social policy and sociology of ageing as well as more popularly that the provision and receipt of care within families is governed by a balance of affect and reciprocity. For instance Bengston et al. (1991: 255), drawing on the work of Gouldner (1960), argue that

> the implied contract of generations calls for the parents to invest a major portion of their resources throughout their adult years in the rearing of children; in old age, the caregiving is expected to be reversed.

In a similar vein, Johnson and his associates (1989: 6) assert that the social contract is analogous to the "implicit contract that exists within families".

In contrast I want to suggest that, as far as the family is concerned, the implied individual-level contract may be a contributory factor in determining the provision of practical care or tending but it is not a *necessary* condition. However, it does feature significantly in the ideological construction of the caring relationship. The main source of these contentions is the research conducted by Qureshi and Walker (1989) in Sheffield among a stratified random sample of just over 300 people aged 75 and over and their principal carer not sharing the same household (see also Walker 1991). The family was, predictably, the main source of care and daughters were the relatives most likely to be providing it. Data from the surveys were used to investigate the importance of affect and reciprocity in determining the supply of care within the family. Neither of them were found to be *necessary* conditions for the provision of practical help.

A simple decision model was created reflecting a traditional western normative preference structure: female relatives would be preferred to male ones, relatives are preferred to non-relatives and so on. In making "decisions" about who provides care, family members very largely behaved as if the hierarchical principles in the model operated in practice, though they may be overruled by situational factors such as the health of prospective carers. Qualitative data indicated that individual family members actually *believed* they had followed the principles implicit in the decision model and also that it reflected their beliefs about what was right.

In most cases, of course, feelings of affect and reciprocity and normative values are mutually reinforcing. However, some insight into the power of these normative obligations, and the fact that they are constructed to some extent *externally* to the caring relationship itself and the life-course processes that preceded it, can be gained by looking at the position of those who provided care despite highly antagonistic individual-level feelings. There were one in six adult children in the carers' study who considered that their relationship with their parent had always been one-sided and who felt no obligation based on intergenerational reciprocity. The motivations of this minority of children who did not think that they owed any debt to their parents, yet still provided the necessary care, are illustrated in this quotation:

> I couldn't stand him but yet I knew it was my duty and no matter what it cost me I would have done that for my own conscience . . . and because of what people say, "Well he's got a daughter and she doesn't do anything for him" . . . I've seen all these articles in the *Star* (local newspaper) I've seen all these pictures of old people and it's been said "Got a son who didn't do anything for them", but nothing is said about what the son or daughter had to put up with to cause them to turn that way. (Qureshi & Walker 1989: 140)

It must be stressed that this sort of comment came from a minority of caring children whose relationship with a parent or parents had been poor over a long period, often as a result of violence and abuse in childhood. In most cases the nature of the caring relationship rests on a delicate balance between reciprocity, affection and duty (Marshall et al. 1987), though in this research few children specifically mentioned love as a reason for helping and were much more likely to refer to duty or obligation.

While the quality of the caring relationship may depend on individual-level factors such as intergenerational reciprocity, its existence owes more to normative constructions. In the first place, choices about who should care for older people are based on rules that derive from stereotyped beliefs about the reciprocal "debts" owed by children to their parents and expectations about appropriate gender roles. Secondly, even though in most instances where care is given, it is clear that people do feel a personalized sense of obligation towards their parents for past help, it is equally clear from the Sheffield research that a significant minority do not share these feelings, yet still feel compelled to help by pressures external to the particular relationship. Indeed in some instances it was evident that intergenerational relationships between family members could be far more difficult and emotionally damaging than other relationships. In these cases the implied intergenerational contract was null and void as far as the carers were concerned because their parent(s) had never opened such a contract in the first place. Thus in some instances care was being provided to older people by female kin in the absence of familial contractual obligations, deriving from any felt need for reciprocity, or affection. Furthermore in some cases care was given despite strong personal antipathy on the part of the carer for the person she was caring for.

The state and intergenerational care

Consideration of precisely how these powerful normative obligations are reproduced requires that the focus of attention is shifted from this brief discussion of microsocial relations back to the macro ones. The state occupies a central role in the social construction of the traditional intergenerational caring relationship and, therefore, in the maintenance of the dominant role of the family, and female kin in particular, in caring for older people. There is not space here to dwell on the impact of the gender division of labour in care (see Finch & Groves 1983, Lewis & Meredith 1988, Qureshi & Walker 1989) our primary concern is with how the division of labour and intergenerational obligations are reproduced socially.

How does the state influence, directly or indirectly, the provision of care by families? A variety of direct methods exists, varying from outright coercion (for example legislation in Canada and Israel that echo the nineteenth-century English Poor Law obligations placed on adult children to support their parents) through to the provision of incentives, such as tax allowances or additional benefits for those caring for dependants. Secondly, the state can influence family help less directly by the way it organizes and provides services to individuals in need and the assumptions it makes about the nature and availability of such assistance in rationing care. Thirdly, the state's general economic and social policies set the framework of material and social conditions within which individual families find themselves. Thus broad welfare policy may help to increase or reduce strains in and around the caring relationship by, for example, the levels of the social security and social services provision it sets. Thus the state may have a direct influence on the quality of intergenerational relations within the family by the sorts of welfare policies it adopts. However, in industrial societies, it is the operation of covert forms of power, particularly at an ideological level, that gives the state its primary influence over the life-world.

In the care of older people outright coercion has rarely proved successful. The idea that the state could compel families to offer love and gratitude to their older parents was given little credence even by the administrators of the English Poor Law. For example they commented, regretfully, on the fact that even the most obvious needs of older people failed to call forth sufficient informal support, despite coercive measures:

if the deficiencies of parental and filial affection are to be supplied by the parish, and the natural motives to the exercise of those virtues are thus to be withdrawn, it may be proper to endeavour to replace them, however imperfectly, by artificial stimulants, and to make fines, distress warrants, or imprisonment act as substitutes for gratitude and love. The attempt however is hardly ever made. (Checkland & Checkland 1974: 115)

Assessing the evidence of attempts by governments over the course of two centuries to impose on families financial responsibility for their relatives Finch (1989: 243) comments:

When government was attempting to impose a version of family responsibilities which people regarded as unreasonable, many responded by developing avoidance strategies: moving to another household, losing touch with their relatives, cheating the system . . . . It seems that it is not in the power of governments straight-forwardly to manipulate what we do for our relatives, let alone what we believe to be proper.

Indeed, if informal care is unwillingly given it loses its special qualities – particularly the intrinsic benefits such as emotional warmth, affection and interest and can no longer claim to be a superior form of care. In fact in this situation it can become rapidly destructive of relationships, inducing resentment and guilt in both giver and receiver.

So, in western societies, the state is very reluctant to intervene directly in the caring relationship, indeed a norm of non-intervention or, at best, minimum intervention may be said to operate. This norm is underpinned by fears that if state help is too easy to obtain it would undermine intergenerational obligations and that this would have serious fiscal implications. This assumption concerning the impact of state provision is well documented in Europe from late Victorian times (Booth 1894, Anderson 1977, Wall 1990) and it appears to be as deeply embedded culturally, if not more so, in the USA (Kreps 1977). It must be emphasized, however, that the persistence of this norm owes nothing to empirical evidence – both historical and contemporary – which has repeatedly come to the opposite conclusion: state support, rather than coercion, can enhance the quality of intergenerational relations (Anderson 1977, Levin et al. 1986, Wall 1990). For example, Wall (1990: 4) points out that in the late nineteenth and early twentieth centuries older people were frequently welcomed into the households of their children because of the Poor Law relief, and later the pensions, they brought with them. A closely related argument is that state welfare provision has resulted in the breakup of the family because there are said to be fewer joint households than in past times. But the simplistic assumption of a linear progression, from pre-industrial times when older people lived with their children to modern time when they live on their own, has been disproved by historical research (Laslett 1965, Wall 1984).

As well as worries concerning the possible abrogation of intergenerational caring responsibilities the reluctance of the state to intervene in the family to provide help and support probably owes something to the fact that the state is a patriarchal state, in that it is dominated both by men and by the ideology of patriarchy (Barrett 1980). This means that the state has an implicit interest in supporting traditional, that is gendered, patterns of caring.

Despite the weight of contrary evidence, health and social care programmes are built on the principle of non-intervention or, at best, minimum intervention. This is not to suggest that there is no state intervention in the care of older people. Of course there is an infrastructure of social service provision even in residual welfare state regimes. But such intervention is usually of a minimum, last resort, kind. For example social services are usually organized on a casualty basis: the provision of home care follows a crisis in the informal caring relationship rather than being allocated at an earlier stage to support this relationship; access to public residential or nursing home care follows hospitalization or carer breakdown. In operating the principle of non-intervention the state is attempting to perpetuate the myth that the family is a private domain. This emphasizes the fact that it is not via direct intervention in the family that the state maintains the primacy of intergenerational obligations, which brings me back to the role of ideology.

In practice the state in all western societies intervenes actively in the family but it does so mainly in the form of ideology rather than by open coercion (Moroney 1976, Donzelot 1979). In particular the state supports the reproduction of the gender division of domestic labour and intergenerational obligations with regard to care and legitimizes these as "normal" or "natural", while at the same time it promotes the myth of the private world of the family. For example in rationing home care in Britain it is common for the proximity of a daughter to be used as a criterion. Social security provision for women who give up paid employment to care for sick or elderly relatives excluded married women until, in 1986, the European Court outlawed this discriminatory practice. The norm of non-intervention in some aspects of the life-world reinforces itself in limiting demands for social services and in ensuring that the family and women in particular perform the two sets of functions essential for social reproduction. On the one hand there is daily reproduction, including the care of sick and elderly family members and, on the other, the intergenerational transmission of values and obligations. In this way the boundaries to the roles of the family and the state are socially constructed not, for the most part, in statute but through the reproduction of "normal" patterns and duties of family life.

At the centre of this process of reproduction is the hegemony of what has been called the ideology of familism (Barrett & McIntosh 1982, Dalley 1988). This is the ideological construction of the individualistic, privatized western family form – with its characteristic gender division of labour and normative belief system concerning intergenerational responsibilities for care. This ideology and particularly its prescriptive norms concerning intergenerational obligations with regard to care is internalized by family members, as we have seen, and even when there is no individual-level contract they still act according to a general sense of duty. Non-conformity to the hegemony of familism is regarded as deviant by other family members and by society (Dalley 1988: 21).

Within this ideology of familism the family is portrayed as a haven from the outside world. Women are located centrally as the providers of nurture and care. They are regarded as "natural" carers and their intergenerational altruism is also seen as "natural". They conform, in this portrayal, to the selflessness and altruism epitomized by the

31

Victorian ideal of women. But, as the research outlined above demonstrates, female kin are under enormous normative pressures to provide care and, therefore, their actions should more correctly be regarded as what Land & Rose (1985) call "compulsory altruism".

Familism and welfare restructuring

It is widely accepted that key aspects of modern welfare state regime were founded, to a considerable extent, on the unpaid domestic labour of women (and on their low paid employment within welfare institutions). Social policies in the realms of social security, health and social care have reflected and reinforced the ideology of familism, for example, by assuming that the family is necessarily the right location for the care of older people and, that, within it, female kin are the most appropriate carers.

As policies to restructure welfare states have developed since the early 1980s the social construction of the natural role of the family in caring for older people and, within the family, the implied contract between the generations, have figured prominently. This is particularly the case in those countries under the influence of neo-liberal ideas, in which the traditional family has a central role. For example, Friedman & Friedman (1980: 135) argue, in the face of the evidence, that in the past

> Children helped their parents out of love and duty. They now contribute to the support of someone else's parents out of compulsion and fear. The earlier transfers strengthened the bonds of the family; the compulsory transfers weaken them.

Or as Margaret Thatcher (1981) put it when she was prime minister:

> . . . it all really starts in the family, because not only is the family the most important means through which we show our care for others. It's the place where each generation learns its responsibilities towards the rest of society. . . . I think the statutory services can only play their part successfully if we don't expect them to do for us things that we could be doing for ourselves.

Under the direct or indirect influence of beliefs such as this, the ideology of familism has been employed by policy-makers to resist increases in public expenditure on the health and social services as a result of the rise in the so-called "burden of dependency". Thus policies, such as "community care", have been presented as preferable alternatives to institutional care but for largely economic reasons, with insufficient resources devoted to them to ensure that a superior quality of care is provided (Walker 1987, 1995). Indeed serious doubt has been cast on the ability of the personal social services to continue functioning without additional resources (Schorr 1992). At the same time the family is expected to play an even greater part in caring for older people even though the research evidence shows that there is little spare capacity for it to do so (Qureshi & Walker 1989).

Just as welfare state restructuring has been part of the driving force behind the imposition of a new pensions contract between the generations, so the old "implied" social contract within the family is being reinforced and used to justify reductions in spending on health and social services. But, as Bengston and his colleagues point out, demographic trends have produced "dramatic changes in intergenerational patterns" within families (Bengston et al. 1991: 3, Bengston 1993). For example it will be increasingly common for families to contain two generations of pensioners and the adult/child pattern of the grandparent and grandchild relationship will be transformed into an adult/adult one (Hagestad 1988). Moreover family members are spending longer periods than previously occupying intergenera-tional family roles. This means that, for women in particular, both the *duration* and the *intensity* of their caring activities will increase, as demographic change is coupled with limitations in spending on support services. The implications of these two sets of antagonistic developments for relations between the generations and also within generations – especially between male and female domestic partners – are likely to be enormous.

In other words the revisions to the social contract currently taking place in pensions, health and social care are on a collision course with the changes underway in generational patterns within families. Unless policies are modified to mesh-in with these changes the result is likely to be increased generational conflict. Specifically, policies with regard to pensions must ensure not only economic security in old age but also continuing solidarity between old and young; while in the field of health and social care the norm of minimum intervention must be abandoned so that care can be shared more effectively between family and state. With a shrinking pool of family carers, increased female participation in the labour market and considerable extensions in family care giving roles, governments will find it more and more difficult to sustain the pretence that families can care for the rising population of very elderly people with only minimal support.

Conclusion

All western countries are either contemplating modifications to the public pensions and health care contracts between age cohorts or they are in the process of being implemented. The main motivation is the wider goal of welfare restructuring that is, in part, a response to the perceived public expenditure "burdens" associated with population ageing. To some extent official concern about population trends is being artificially amplified as an economic-demographic imperative to legitimize the rewriting of the social contract and more general restructuring. But the pace of change in the introduction of a new social contract differs significantly between countries depending on the ideology currently holding sway. Britain, under neo-liberal inspired policies, has already radically altered its social contract, whereas in Germany the perpetuation of a solidaristic consensus on the welfare state has meant that, so far, the reforms are more modest and the timetable more relaxed. In Britain too the health and personal social services components of the social contract are also being revised radically and the impact of these changes on older people has already attracted severe criticism (Henwood 1992, Schorr 1992, Walker 1995).

"Intergenerational equity" rhetoric concerning "greedy elders" has proved to be something of a red herring in this process of change. It has been confined very largely to the USA with the vast majority of European countries and even the USA's close neighbour Canada remaining immune. Moreover despite dire predictions and ample rhetoric, particularly in the USA, there is no actual evidence of overt age cohort conflicts. However, the processes of fashioning a new generational contract may themselves create the conditions for *both* intergenerational and age cohort conflicts. The modifications of the social contract underway in western society consist of important institutional reforms in the fields of pensions, health care and social care; reforms that could have far reaching effects on future age cohort relations. For example, since the early 1980s in Britain the emphasis on individual responsibility and the switch from public to personal pensions may encourage future cohorts to think selfishly more in terms of their own life-cycle rather than solidaristically (Bengston et al. 1991: 270, Walker 1994). This may, in turn, weaken social integration between age cohorts. Similarly the reduction in the rights of older relatives to NHS care and the attempts to increase the role of the family in the care of older people will result in more economic pressures falling on the family and greater caring responsibilities falling on female kin. This has all the pent-up potential of a pressure-cooker to create new conflicts both between carers and older relatives and within the carer's own nuclear family.

As Bengston (1993) has pointed out, in the USA the consequences of the current generational watershed may be either increased conflict between age cohorts or increased solidarity. The main argument of this chapter has been that whether the twenty-first century holds the prospect of conflict or consensus is primarily a matter of social and economic policy rather than of any properties inherent in age cohorts themselves. The precise outcome depends on the interaction of macro- and micro-level factors. Certainly age-group conflicts have the potential for greater prominence in the decades to come, but the key question is how far will the societal context within which these cohorts experience ageing be conducive to conflict or solidarity? At the present time, as far as Britain is concerned, it appears that economic and social policies aimed at creating new contracts between age cohorts in the realms of pensions, health and social care are likely to increase the potential for both intercohort and intergenerational conflict. Yet there is no evidence that policy makers (nor mainstream social science) have begun to take seriously this momentous issue.

Notes

1. The main elements of welfare state restructuring have been: reductions in social expenditure, usually in comparison with rising need or inflation; recommodification, in the form of either direct privatization or the extension of market principles within the state sector; the replacement of universal benefits with selective ones; tax reductions and incentives to use private welfare; substitution of voluntary and private welfare for public provision; increasing the role of the informal sector in care; and centralization of resource control coupled with the decentralization of operational responsibility. It is the combination of these policies that has enabled neo-liberal governments, such as those of Britain and New Zealand, to tightly control resource distribution through the welfare state and begin to lower public expectations and, thereby, to assist

accumulation yet also tackle the legitimation crisis (Shirley 1990, Walker 1990c).

2. It is *not* being argued that actors are the creatures of ideology. But rather that, analytically speaking, ideology plays a crucial role in mediating between the external social system and the internal environment of individual actors. In doing so it can exert a powerful influence over action from both spheres, that is, by being internalized on the one hand and reflected in external social relations and networks on the other. The precise degree of influence will depend on a range of factors, including the strength and legitimacy of the ideology in question and the particular situational constraints on action.

CHAPTER 2

Intergenerational relationships past and present

Richard Wall

Introduction

There is a strong presumption that within western Europe, kinship ties, including those between the elderly and their children, have weakened over the course of time. Individual instances of the neglect of the elderly by their close kin can certainly be found but these can be documented for societies in the past as well as for those in the present, while it is possible to counter every case of wilful neglect with another demonstrating support, financial, social or both (Laslett 1989: 127, 132). At a more general level both Fréderic Le Play and Charles Booth collected data on mid-nineteenth-century Europe and late-nineteenth-century England and Wales respectively that demonstrated that the majority of the elderly in the societies studied were not financially dependent on their children (summarized in Wall 1992). Wealth more often passed down the generational chain rather than up, even during the life-time of those parents. There is also evidence, admittedly only from England, that the proportion of married children living within five miles of their parents and therefore close enough to permit regular contact, has not altered between the late eighteenth and mid-twentieth centuries (Wall 1992: 73).

The identification of the "old"

It is conventional to take the age of 65 as marking the point of entry into old age. The age group 65–74 are considered as the "young old" or the "golden oldies" and all those over 75 as the "old old". Yet there are other important factors such as retirement or semi-retirement, the age from which the state provides pensions (currently in Britain from age 65 for men and from age 60 for women), the issue of deteriorating health and even the age of one's partner that may alternatively hasten or retard the transition into old age for a given individual. In the past, too, it seems likely that there was considerable variability between one individual and another in the age at which they felt themselves to be old or were viewed as old by their neighbours. Yet images of a stereotyped old age can also be found for past societies, ranging from the biblical three score years and ten as being the natural span of life to artists' impressions of the life-cycle that see the high point of life reached between the ages of 50 and 59. Such representations of the life-cycle present the image of a relatively benign early old age followed by a long period of increasing decrepitude: see Figure 2.1 (Hazelzet 1990).

The necessity of balancing the stages coming early and late in the life-cycle within the compass of the one picture may well in this case have forced an overly long representation of the period of life spent in old age. The reality for the majority of the inhabitants of past societies would have been quite different, even for the fortunate few who had survived through into their early sixties. For example, censuses of six rural populations all dating from before 1800 indicate out of a total female population of 2,358, there were just 76 women aged 60–64, no more than 31 aged 70–74 and only 3 over the age of 85. This population moreover is likely to have enjoyed among the highest life expectancy of any pre-industrial population as geographical remoteness and less crowding than in the towns reduced the incidence of infectious disease (Wrigley & Schofield 1983: 178). Secondly, the female rather than the male population has been selected for illustrative purposes as in the past women in western societies generally outlived men for a number of reasons whose precise impact is difficult to measure, although differences in life-style seem clearly to have been of greater relevance than any innate biological advantage enjoyed over men (Johanson 1991).

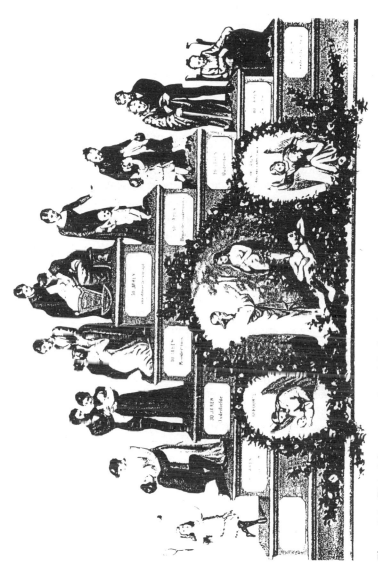

Figure 2.1 Pictorial representation of the female life-cycle. Reproduced by kind permission of the Museum Voor Volkskunde, Bruges, Belgium.

The old, therefore, were a rarity in the past but it does not necessarily follow that the family and household patterns of the fortunate few who did reach old age diverged significantly from those of the elderly in the present day developed world when most people live on into old age. To establish just how different these patterns were is the first objective of the present chapter. The common expectation is that the elderly in the past would have lived in complex households formed around the families of their married children. In fact as far as pre-industrial England is concerned, this has been shown to be an idealized misrepresentation of the past, yet one that is particularly enduring (cf. Laslett 1989). The second aim of the chapter is to use the information on living arrangements across the life-cycle to comment on the extent to which the family and household patterns of those individuals who survived to old age diverged radically from those of younger people in the same societies. In particular, attention will be paid to the age from which the family patterns associated with old age, whether living alone or other arrangements, first exhibit a marked upward trend, as indicating the point from when certain elements within the population first began to experience some of the problems associated with "classic" old age. Such persons can be considered as "old before their time" as far as their family and household patterns are concerned even though they might not have thought of themselves, or been seen by others, as belonging to the population of the elderly. As one measure of the ageing process it has to be viewed in conjunction with other indications of old age, notably a "socially recognized" old age. Even for populations in the past, a number of such indications are available. Reference has already been made to the pictorial representations of the life-cycle and in due course another indicator will be used, the point in the life-cycle after which a sharp increase can be observed in the proportion of older adults residing in institutions.

Changes in the living arrangements of persons aged 65+ between pre-industrial times and the present day

The classification of living arrangements that it has been decided to adopt follows closely the classifications of relationships within households implemented by Statistics Canada and the Central Statistics Office of Ireland as part of their census programme of the 1970s and

1980s (Central Statistics Office, Dublin 1983; Statistics Canada 1987). The essence of the classification is the identification of a hierarchy of relationships within the household, beginning with the couple and then proceeding in turn to identify persons with at least one co-resident never-married child, persons who lived with relatives other than their spouse or never-married child, persons who lived with non-related people only and, finally, persons who lived alone. Couples and parents with their never-married children constitute families. All others are considered as living outside families. In addition for the purpose of this chapter, couples include both *de facto* (co-habiting) couples and the married and never-married children can be of any age. The strength of the classification lies in its identification of core relationships, couples and parent and child. One weakness is that the category "other relatives" is rather heterogenous. For example, from the perspective of those elderly persons who did not belong to a family (as defined), their relatives could include married, divorced or widowed children as well as siblings (married or unmarried) or more distant relatives. However, in reality most of these "other relatives" would have been married children, because living with other types of relatives in the absence of children is known to be rare in the English experience (Wall 1992: 68–9).

For the purposes of illustrating the change in living arrangements over the course of time, five periods have been selected (Table 2.1). The first, covering the two centuries from the end of the sixteenth century, is unsatisfactorily broad. However, there is no alternative but to group the data from the various populations given the small number of the surviving censuses from this period that specify the ages and the relationships of members of the household, and given that so few of the inhabitants reached the age of 65. A useful division, however, can be made between a group of smaller, largely rural populations (although less than one-fifth of the heads of household were farmers) and the city of Lichfield, enumerated in 1692, and which represented a far less healthy environment (Fiennes cited in Morris 1947: 114).

Anonymized data from the censuses of 1891 and 1921 for 53 clusters of enumeration districts provide further perspectives on the living arrangements of the elderly. For the purposes of presentation, the data from all these populations have been pooled. Space constraints preclude an extended account of the nature of the data (for further details see Garrett & Reid 1994, Wall 1994) but it should be noted that the clusters do not constitute a random sample of the national population but

Table 2.1 Living arrangements of persons aged 65+: England and Wales, sixteenth to twentieth centuries.

Living arrangements	Rural English populations before 1800[a]	Lichfield 1692	Lichfield 1891[b]	England and Wales 1921[b]	England and Wales 1971[c]	England and Wales 1981[c]
Males						
Living alone	2	5	5	6	13	17
Non-relatives only	11	8	13	10	4	3
Spouse (with/ without others)	58	68	57	57	73	73
Lone parent with never-married child	16	16	10	12	3	2
Other relatives only	14	3	15	15	7	5
Total[d]	100	100	100	100	100	100
N	102	38	1,699	2,620	24,836	30,175
Females						
Living alone	15	17	11	11	36	42
Non-relatives only	17	32	14	11	5	3
Spouse (with/ without others)	40	23	30	32	36	38
Lone parent with never married child	6	20	18	20	7	6
Other relatives only	23	9	28	26	15	11
Total[d]	100	100	100	100	100	100
N	102	66	2,121	3,295	38,361	45,123

a. Derived from an analysis of the censuses of Ealing (Middlesex) in 1599, Chilvers Coton (Warwickshire) in 1684, Wetherby (Yorkshire) in 1776, Wembworthy (Devon) in 1779, Corfe Castle (Dorset) in 1790 and Ardleigh (Essex) in 1796.
b. Anonymized data from census returns for parts of the following areas: Abergavenny (Monmouthshire), Axminster (Devon), Banbury (Oxford-shire), Bethnal Green (London), Bolton (Lancashire), Earsdon (Northumberland), Morland (Westmorland), Pinner (Middlesex), Saffron Walden (Essex), Stoke (Staffordshire), Swansea (Glamorgan), Walthamstow (Essex) and the city of York.
c. Calculated from the national samples of the English and Welsh populations taken by the Office of Population Censuses and Surveys for the purpose of the Longitudinal Study.
d. Includes a few cases of never-married persons aged 65+ living with a parent.

were drawn from 13 "places", selected principally because of their geographical and economic diversity. The range of variation from place to place in household and family patterns is therefore likely to be large. Nevertheless, when taken as a group, the characteristics of these populations in terms of age structure and marital status distributions deviate surprisingly little from those of the national population. No comparisons of course can be made of their family and household structure as no nationwide data are available for this period.

The final two periods effectively chose themselves: 1971 and 1981 are the latest censuses currently available. For analysis purposes, use has been made of the 1 per cent cross sections of the population taken for the purposes of the Longitudinal Study. These censuses permit the pace of change in residence patterns since the 1970s to be gauged as well as the extent of change since 1921. The intervening gap is, admittedly, uncomfortably large, as is that between the pre-industrial period and the end of the nineteenth century, but both can be closed to some extent by reference to more summary measures of the composition of households derived from both census and survey sources (for the nineteenth century see Anderson 1990 and for the twentieth, Wall 1992).

It is now time to consider the characteristic living arrangements of persons aged 65+ over the course of the centuries. Focusing first on the living arrangements of elderly men it will be seen from Table 2.1 that even in pre-industrial times there were men of this age who lived on their own. A greater proportion resided only with non-relatives and from one perspective might be thought of as living on their own, as in such a situation it is likely that they were budgeting separately from other members of the household. The most frequently encountered living arrangement, however, was that a man over the age of 65 would still have his wife resident in the household. More than half of all such men were in this situation in the pre-industrial rural populations and more than two-thirds of those in Lichfield in 1692. This naturally left only a minority, under one-fifth in each case, who lived either as lone parents with never-married children or with other relatives, principally married children.

The examination of the changes that have occurred in the living arrangements of older men since pre-industrial times shows very little sign of change by the end of the nineteenth century or even by 1921. The one clear difference was that in 1891 and 1921 fewer men lived as a lone parent with a never-married child. By 1971, on the other hand, the

residence patterns of the elderly men look quite different with substantial rises in the percentage of men over the age of 65 living alone
and compensatory declines in the percentages of such men living with
non-relatives only, with never-married children or with other relatives. The decline in the percentage living as lone parents with their
never-married children has been particularly marked, with demographic factors prominent in bringing about the changes. The sustained fall in fertility that occurred in the earlier part of the twentieth
century, the alteration in the timing of births that has resulted in the
concentration of child-bearing into the years immediately following
marriage and the increased proportion of the population who by the
middle years of the twentieth century would eventually marry, have
all lessened the probability that persons entering old age would still
have never-married children resident in their households. By contrast,
the rise in the proportion of men over the age of 65 who live alone
seems more likely to be economic in origin, reflecting the increased
standard of living of the population that makes it easier to provide
smaller housing units that can be clearly seen as being occupied by
independent households. In the past, the vast majority of the elderly
who lived with non-relatives were probably semi-independent, not
residentially independent but economically independent, and were
therefore not recorded as forming their own households. Yet it is interesting that if the household is defined as an economic rather than as a
residence unit, in other words if the categories of men living alone and
with non-relatives are combined, then the change in living arrangements from pre-industrial times through to the late twentieth century
appears much less dramatic with approximately 13 per cent of men
over the age of 65 "living independently" in rural pre-industrial
England, 18 per cent in 1891, and 16 per cent in 1921 compared with 17
per cent in 1971 and 20 per cent in 1981.

One other change has been the rise since pre-industrial times from
58 per cent (in the rural populations) to 73 per cent of men over the age
of 65 who were still married. That this percentage was as high as it was
in the pre-industrial population, despite the much higher mortality,
again owes much to demographic factors. In the past, as today, women
on average outlived men and were in any case younger than their
spouse on average at marriage (and remarriage). It is therefore not surprising that those men who did reach old age might still have their
spouse resident in their household. However, in addition the
unbalanced sex ratio in the adult population (relatively more women),

and the greater economic power of the men, certainly gave the widower more chance to remarry than the widow.

The living arrangements of the women over the age of 65 look rather different (Table 2.1). As already indicated rather fewer women than men from this age group still had a co-resident spouse, and higher proportions of elderly women lived alone, or with other relatives, these for the most part being their married children. In pre-industrial rural England, however, the most frequently encountered situation was still that of co-resident spouse, but there were sizeable minorities of women over the age of 65 living alone or with non-relatives only (under one-fifth in each case) or with other relatives (over one-fifth). Living as a lone parent with a never-married child was, in pre-industrial rural England, considerably rarer: only 6 per cent of such women did so.

By the end of the nineteenth century, this pattern of living arrangements had altered considerably, and certainly to a greater extent than had the residence patterns of elderly men. The percentage of women over the age of 65 who lived alone, with non-relatives only or with a spouse had all fallen dramatically (and in the case of co-residence with non-relatives was to fall further by 1921) while the percentage living with other relatives had risen considerably, as had the percentage living with never-married children, at least when compared with the situation of women from the rural pre-industrial populations. At the end of the nineteenth century it would appear that elderly women were more likely to have been drawing on the social (and presumably the financial) support of their children, with little sign of further change before 1921 (see Ruggles 1987 on the rise of the extended family during the nineteenth century).

The situation in the late twentieth century, however, differs again with a marked rise in the proportion of elderly women living alone, something of a recovery in the proportion who resided with a spouse, and marked falls in the proportion residing as lone parents with never-married children or with other relatives. As in the case of men, these changes can be seen as being in part furthered by demographic and in part by economic change, although the precise mix of factors is somewhat different. For women the rise in the proportion living alone, for example, is occasioned not only by the improvement in living standards that has allowed a higher proportion of the population to live independently, but also through the fact that female life expectancy has increased faster than male life expectancy, leaving many women spending a long period of time as widows and therefore at risk of living alone. It is for this reason, too, that the proportion of women over the age of 65 who are married was still in 1981 below that recorded for those women who survived into old age in pre-industrial rural England.

The final remarks on Table 2.1 will be reserved for a few comments on the differences between the living arrangements of elderly men and women in the rural pre-industrial populations and those of the elderly in the city of Lichfield in 1692. Some differences can certainly be expected. Lichfield was undoubtedly much more unhealthy (Morris 1947) but it also differed socially and economically because of its function as a regional centre on a major route to the north-west of England and with a number of relatively wealthy people congregating around the cathedral and, in the process, bringing much additional trade to the town. The principal feature of the living arrangements of the elderly in Lichfield that distinguished them from those of the elderly in the rural populations was, for both men and women, the much reduced frequency of living with other relatives and, for women, the increased incidence of living either with non-relatives only or as a lone parent with a never-married child. It is conceivable that the nature of urban housing permitted a greater degree of subdivision of property than was possible in the rural area. On the other hand it may be that the poverty of some sections of Lichfield's population forced such a subdivision or that there was a real shortage of housing at a suitable price. At this distance it is difficult to be sure, although Lichfield was far from uniformly prosperous as the proportion of exemptions from payment of the hearth tax shows (William Salt Archaeological Society 1921: 159). Whatever the actual explanation may be, at least the impact on the living arrangements of the elderly in Lichfield is clear enough. There is also another major difference in that the proportion of men over the age of 65 still living with a spouse is considerably in excess of that prevailing in the rural populations while the reverse applies in the case of elderly women. Again, unfortunately, it is not possible to establish the pattern of causation with any degree of certainty but it seems likely that older men profited from their favourable position in the marriage market, evidence for which comes from the unbalanced sex ratio of the adult population, to remarry in the event of the death of their spouse. The excess of women in the population was itself occasioned by both the different migration patterns of men and women affecting primarily the age range 20–35 (more men moving out of Lichfield and more women moving in) and by differential life expectancy, the impact of which only becomes clearly visible after the age of 55.

The late sixties as a turning point in the life-cycle

The same classification scheme of living arrangements will now be used to address the second major theme of this chapter: the extent to which the family and household patterns of those over the age of 65 diverged from those who had yet to reach, and perhaps would never reach, this classic threshold into old age. Tables 2.2–2.5 indicate how many men and women in five year age groups from 45 through to 85+ lived alone, with non-relatives only, with relatives other than a spouse or unmarried child, as a lone parent with an unmarried child, or were co-resident with their spouse. The populations covered are four out of the five that have already been under consideration, pre-industrial rural England before 1800, the thirteen local populations from England and Wales in 1891 and 1921, and the national sample of individuals from the census of England and Wales of 1981. Membership of a family is also defined as before: that it includes both married and *de facto* couples (where the latter can be identified) and parents with their unmarried children.

Table 2.2 covers the situation in rural pre-industrial England. As expected, the vast majority of middle-aged men and women lived with a spouse, whereas in old age this was much less likely particularly in the case of women. What is interesting, however, is that there was one particular residence pattern that predominated in old age, or even in extreme old age (among persons over the age of 75). There was therefore no residence pattern that could be clearly associated with old age. Half of the few elderly men who survived into their early eighties were still married or had been able to remarry while the remainder lived either with unmarried children or other relatives, and occasionally with non-relatives only. Very rarely did they live alone. Moreover, the residence patterns of elderly women were characterized by an even greater degree of diversity with considerable numbers living with relatives in the absence of a spouse and child, only with non-relatives, or alone. Nor is there sign, either for men or women, of a more marked change in residence patterns between the early and late sixties than occurred between any other five year age

47

Table 2.2 Living arrangements during middle and old age: English rural populations before 1800.

Age group	Alone	Non-relatives only	With relatives (no spouse or unmarried child)	Lone parent and unmarried child	With spouse	N
Males						
45–9	3	10	0	4	82	79
50–4	0	10	4	6	81	114
55–9	0	9	4	9	79	57
60–4	4	12	3	15	67	96
65–9	0	15	7	17	61	41
70–4	6	7	10	10	68	31
75–9	0	7	14	29	50	14
80–4	0	0	30	20	50	10
85+	0	33	50	0	17	6
Females						
45–9	3	4	4	14	72	90
50–4	2	7	7	16	67	123
55–9	2	9	2	11	77	57
60–4	7	17	7	18	51	76
65–9	18	11	18	9	43	44
70–4	10	16	19	3	52	31
75–9	12	24	29	0	35	17
80–4	14	43	29	14	0	7
85+	33	0	67	0	0	3

Note: A few unmarried children aged 45+ and resident with a parent are included in the total but are not shown separately. Percentages may not sum to 100 due to rounding.
Source: See Table 2.1

groups. Indeed, there was considerably less change during the sixties than either earlier or in the relative frequency of co-residence with a spouse, the dominant residence pattern of middle age.

In certain respects little had changed by the end of the nineteenth century (see Table 2.3). There is, for example, no sign of a major transformation in residence patterns as people passed through their sixties, and in old age, and extreme old age a variety of living arrangements were possible for both men and women. There was, however, one important change in that co-residence with "other" relatives, most of whom would have been married children, had become relatively more important. In 1891 this was the predominant living arrangement of women over the age of 75, and even for men over this age, it was

Table 2.3 Living arrangements during middle and old age: England and Wales 1891.

Age group	Alone	Non-relatives only	With relatives (no spouse or unmarried child)	Lone parent and unmarried child	With spouse	N
Males						
45–9	1	7	3	6	81	1,906
50–4	2	11	3	6	78	1,539
55–9	3	8	4	8	76	1,198
60–4	3	10	8	9	70	1,017
65–9	4	11	9	10	66	736
70–4	5	12	14	10	58	515
75–9	6	14	28	9	44	298
80–4	6	19	28	12	35	95
85+	11	18	20	13	35	55
Females						
45–9	2	6	5	14	71	1,919
50–4	3	6	8	17	63	1,727
55–9	3	8	9	19	61	1,323
60–4	6	9	15	19	51	1,181
65–9	9	12	20	19	39	905
70–4	12	13	29	17	29	652
75–9	14	16	34	16	20	351
80–4	10	16	49	15	9	136
85+	16	18	42	18	6	77

Note: Excludes persons resident in institutions and visitors. A few unmarried children aged 45+ and resident with a parent are included in the total but are not shown separately. Percentages may not sum to 100 due to rounding.
Sources: See Table 2.1

the most frequently encountered arrangement apart from co-residence with a spouse. The elderly at the end of the nineteenth century therefore experienced both a diversity in living arrangements and one particular residence pattern, co-residence with relatives other than spouse and unmarried child, which could be considered as typically associated with old age, even though it never represented the experience of the majority in any of the five year age groups.

Thirty years later, co-residence with "other" relatives was still the most common residence pattern for women over the age of 75, and the second most important pattern for very old men (see Table 2.4). Among older women, however, it had lost a little of its earlier popularity, largely due to the fact that co-residence with unmarried children

Table 2.4 Living arrangements during middle and old age: England and Wales 1921.

Age group	Alone	Non-relatives only	With relatives (no spouse or unmarried child)	Lone parent and unmarried child	With spouse	N
Males						
45–9	1	7	4	4	81	3,147
50–4	2	8	6	6	77	2,555
55–9	2	9	6	6	77	2,158
60–4	4	8	8	7	73	1,672
65–9	6	10	10	11	64	1,214
70–4	5	10	16	10	59	728
75–9	7	10	20	18	44	445
80–4	12	13	24	13	37	173
85+	8	18	35	15	23	60
Females						
45–9	2	6	7	9	71	3,209
50–4	3	7	8	12	67	2,698
55–9	4	7	10	15	63	2,244
60–4	6	8	16	17	53	1,822
65–9	8	10	20	19	42	1,419
70–4	12	10	27	17	33	885
75–9	12	12	35	21	19	609
80–4	16	13	35	24	12	260
85+	14	13	36	27	10	122

Notes: Excludes persons resident in institutions and visitors. A few unmarried children aged 45+ and resident with a parent are included in the total but are not shown separately. Percentages may not sum to 100 due to rounding.
Sources: See Table 2.1

had become relatively more important. The principal features of the residence patterns of the elderly in 1921, therefore, were, as was the case in earlier times, both diversity and the absence of any significant change involving people in their sixties.

The residence patterns of the middle aged and elderly in 1981, on the other hand, differed markedly from those of earlier times in that there is considerably less diversity (Table 2.5). Just two types of living arrangements, co-residence with a spouse and living alone, represented the situation of more than nine out of ten men and eight out of ten women between the ages of 65 and 74 and of more than eight out of ten men (and seven out of ten women) in their early eighties. By

Table 2.5 Living arrangements during middle and old age: England and Wales 1981.

Age group	Alone	Non-relatives only	With relatives (no spouse or unmarried child)	Lone parent and unmarried child	With spouse	N
Males						
45–9	5	3	2	3	84	14,924
50–4	6	3	3	3	83	15,129
55–9	8	3	3	2	84	14,907
60–4	9	3	3	2	83	12,847
65–9	12	3	3	2	80	11,884
70–4	17	3	4	2	75	9,100
75–9	20	4	6	2	69	5,553
80–4	28	4	9	4	55	2,529
85+	32	6	16	5	41	1,109
Females						
45–9	4	2	1	8	83	17,784
50–4	7	2	2	7	80	15,158
55–9	11	2	3	6	76	15,997
60–4	19	3	5	5	67	14,365
65–9	30	3	6	5	56	14,513
70–4	40	3	9	5	43	12,442
75–9	51	3	12	6	28	9,434
80–4	55	4	17	7	17	5,498
85+	51	5	26	10	7	3,236

Notes: Excludes persons resident in institutions and visitors. A few unmarried children aged 45+ and resident with a parent are included in the total but are not shown separately. Percentages may not sum to 100 due to rounding.
Sources: See Table 2.1

1981, living alone when elderly had come into greater prominence, and by implication, was more closely associated with old age than had been the case at the end of the nineteenth century as regards co-residence with other relatives. Yet some features of the residence patterns of earlier times survived even in 1981, notably that the marked decline in the frequency of co-residence with a spouse, the dominant residential arrangement of middle age, occurred when men and women reached their seventies, and not earlier.

Alternative transition points into old age

The pattern of living arrangements across the different age groups has been set out above in some detail in order to emphasize the degree of variability that is dependent on age and gender within a given population. It is clear that there was no set path into old age involving changes to the patterns of family life. Some individuals had already adopted living arrangements typically associated with old age before they had reached the age of 50, while others retained their membership of a family group through into extreme old age. Certainly there are few signs of a major shift in family patterns occurring during the late sixties, the period in life classically associated with old age, in any of the time periods (pre-industrial, nineteenth century and early and late twentieth century) that have been under investigation. Moreover, a much greater degree of variability would have been suggested had there been longitudinal data available to facilitate calculation of the flows of people into and out of particular types of family and household.

Of course, as mentioned above, the old and the not so old can be differentiated in other ways than in terms of their family patterns, through their presence or absence from the labour market, their health status or, formally, through the receipt of a pension, however inadequate an income that might give them. Some of these events could very well indicate a sharper transition into old age although one that need not necessarily take place at the age of 65 or indeed at the current age in Britain for the award of a state pension (65 for men and 60 for women). In nineteenth-century England, retirement from employment at a set age was an option available only for the privileged few while for the majority, retirement, or partial retirement to a less skilled job or intermittent work, might well ensue following a period of temporary ill health later in life. In such cases the assistance of the Poor Law might be required and would be provided if real need could be proved. Only a few persons, however, received a regular pension from the Poor Law authorities in the nineteenth century before they reached the age of 70 (Robin 1990: 196). Yet whatever the timing of these transitions and however sharp they may have been, for those who had been fortunate enough to keep their core family intact the presence of members of the immediate family circle is likely to have softened the severity of other breaks in the life-course that disrupted previous life-patterns.

For a number of older persons, however, there was no family or only inadequate support available from the family, and another indicator of the social recognition of old age is the age from which increasing proportions of older people entered institutions, either because it was felt they were unable to manage their own households or because they posed too great a burden on the surviving members of their family. Such institutions would include the alms-houses, "hospitals" for the reception of the elderly poor and "town houses" of pre-industrial times, the workhouses of the eighteenth, nineteenth and early twentieth centuries and the nursing and old peoples' homes of the present day. Age on entering into such institutions was also extremely variable, and does not seem to have been tied to the achievement of a particular age. For example, there were some "hospital men" in Lichfield in 1692 who were still in their early fifties, although institutionalization became the common experience, indeed virtually the universal experience only, for the handful of men who were aged over 75. The age range of the "hospital women" of Lichfield was also extremely broad although not as broad as that for the men, in that none of the women was younger than 55. Independent of age, lower proportions of women than of men were lodged in the hospital although there is the same marked increase in the proportion of women institutionalized over the age of 75 that was noted for the men. Interestingly it is after the age of 75 that there is a marked increase in the proportion of the population resident in institutions in England and Wales in 1981 (Wall 1989). One major change, however, is that in 1981 much larger proportions of women than of men are resident in institutions, particularly in the highest age groups (80+). This is the reverse of the situation in Lichfield in 1692 and higher proportions of elderly men than elderly women were also resident in the Ardleigh workhouse in 1796, the only one of the rural populations with its own workhouse.

Undoubtedly, considerable care needs to be taken in the evaluation of the results. The evidential base for the pre-industrial period is slim and it was necessary to infer age of entry into an institution from the age distribution of the residents, given the absence of more direct information (for one historical population with better information see Van der Veen & Van Poppel 1992: 200). Nevertheless enough evidence has hopefully been produced to confirm there were a number of different "transition points" into old age, which could be reached at a variety of ages.

Conclusion

Although there is therefore no one age that rigidly marks off the point of entry into old age, it is still important to determine the character of resident familial support that would be available to those over the age of 65 in case of need and how it has changed over the course of time. The major feature, without any doubt, is the high proportion of men with a co-resident spouse even in extreme old age. For example, in pre-industrial rural England half of all men who survived into the late seventies and early eighties were still married. In 1891 and 1921 many fewer of this age were still married, but still over four in ten of those aged 75–79 and over one-third of those aged 80–84. By 1981 this situation had reversed itself to such an extent that higher proportions of older men were married than had been the case in rural pre-industrial England. It follows that in 1981, as in pre-industrial times, primary care of the older man is most likely to have fallen to his wife, health permitting, whereas at the end of the nineteenth and in the early twentieth centuries, more children, married and unmarried, will have shouldered this responsibility.

Other residence patterns to experience change include the proportion of older men living as lone parents with their never-married children that declined between pre-industrial times and 1891, then rose between 1891 and 1921 only to decline again by 1981. The proportion living with other relatives, principally married children, rose between pre-industrial times and 1891, and then more or less stabilized between 1891 and 1921 before declining sharply. However, the fact that the decline has been proportionately less marked for men over the age of 85 than for men in their sixties and seventies, implies that even in 1981 when care was most likely to be needed, it might in some cases be supplied by a resident member of the family other than the spouse or unmarried child. Finally, the proportions living alone have risen over the course of time although more steeply since the 1960s (Wall 1992), while the proportions living only with non-relatives have decreased, at least since 1891.

Over the course of time many of the living arrangements of older women have altered more dramatically than have those of older men with a much higher proportion of older women in the late nineteenth century and in 1921 living with their never-married children or other relatives (most of them married children) than in either earlier or later times. In all periods, however, it is the case that the closest resident

54

relative of the older women would in a greater proportion of cases be a child, ever or never married, whereas for men this would more likely be their spouse.

The principal feature of the living arrangements of older women in 1981 is the much higher proportion who lived on their own, a trend again induced in part by demographic changes and in part by improvements in the standard of living, with little left for the effect of changes in family values. Indeed, in certain cases a reverse relationship may have operated, for example, the decline in the frequency of co-residence with non-relatives may have induced a greater distrust of "strangers". For those who were not members of the core family, the changes since pre-industrial times have undoubtedly been considerable with an increasing tendency for residential independence, the maintenance of physically separate households, to complement economic independence. On the other hand, it is from a small select group of relatives that support, social or financial, was likely to come if needed and this fact has not altered between the England in the past and the England of the 1990s.

CHAPTER 3

Does Britain have a
welfare generation?

John Hills[1]

Introduction

Much of what the welfare state does is to redistribute income across
people's own life-cycles, rather than redistributing between different
individuals, if one examines its effects over complete life-times
(Falkingham & Hills 1995). Such redistribution could, in principle, be
achieved in two ways. One would be enforced contributions into a
fund that would be invested on its contributors' behalf and drawn on
when needed – much in the way that private sector pension schemes
in fact operate. The second is what has actually occurred in Britain:
welfare services like education, health care and social security are
financed on a "Pay As You Go" basis, using the national insurance
contributions and tax payments drawn (largely) from the current
working generation to pay for the benefits going (largely) to the non-
working generations.

In a steady state, the outcome of these two alternatives might, under
certain conditions, be much the same in terms of the payments into the
system made by each generation, and the amounts each would receive
from it, although outcomes would not necessarily be the same in terms
of the nation's stock of capital, savings rates, and so on.

However, looking back over the twentieth century, the British
welfare state cannot be described as having been in a steady state.
Public spending in Britain on education, health and social security
rose as a percentage of national income from less than 10 per cent for
most of the pre-war period to 20 per cent or more by the mid-1970s. In
such a situation, different generations may easily be being treated

in ways that are more or less favourable than the treatment of others.

Since the late 1980s demographers and economic historians have started to examine the scale of transfers resulting from the operations of the welfare state between actual generations or age cohorts. This analysis has led to some striking conclusions:

> Seen from a cohort perspective, not only the ups and downs of fertility in the twentieth century but also the workings of social security have created considerable injustices between different generations. If perceived as such, this injustice between the generations could foster discontent with future social policies and, finally, undermine the "implicit contract" between generations on which the welfare state is based. (Johnson et al. 1989: 1)

In his analysis of the New Zealand welfare state, Thomson (1991: 1) puts his findings starkly:

> In New Zealand the big winners in this have been the "welfare generation" – those born between about 1920 and 1945. Throughout their lives they will make contributions that cover only a fraction of their benefits. For their successors the reverse is true, and the question now is whether such a welfare state has a future.

He also suggests that this finding is not unique to one country:

> The timing and pace of welfare expansion will have created different generational imbalances in each modern state, yet the similarities are also striking. Analysis . . . suggests a comparable erection of youth-states in the early post-war years in most developed nations. (Thomson 1989: 39)

This is clearly an important issue. If the welfare state is creating generations that are systematically losing from current arrangements, there certainly may be implications for the future of the welfare state in its current form. Already in the USA there has been a pressure group, Americans for Generational Equity (AGE), which proposes cuts in transfers to the elderly on the grounds that they are no longer poor by comparison with the young (Johnson & Falkingham 1992: 132) By the same token, *changes* to existing arrangements that have the effect, for instance, of reducing the expected receipts of certain generations when they reach old age, might create imbalances that did not exist before, and turn generations who expected to "break-even" in some sense into net losers. Political conflict between generations over who gets what out of the welfare state and over who pays for it may come to be added to the existing conflicts between rich and poor, men and women, South and North, and so on (see Ch. 1).

However, the arguments are not clear cut. First, the use of Pay As You Go funding does not of itself prove that intergenerational inequity exists, as is explored below. Secondly, even if inequity does exist in some countries, it may not in others. Indeed, Johnson & Falkingham (1988b: 144) suggest that, in Britain,

> . . . the welfare system has been remarkably neutral in its treat-
> ment of the young and the old, and in this respect recent trends
> in Britain have clearly been different from those perceived by
> Preston for the US and Thomson for New Zealand.

Thirdly, it is not clear that the kinds of analyses used to reach the conclusions of intergenerational inequity deployed by Thomson and others prove their case. It may be true that certain forms of welfare provision that used to favour the young have been cut back, while others that favour the old have been increased. But this does not, of itself, prove that there has been a net transfer between particular generations. That depends on exactly which age cohorts have benefited when from each part of social spending, and, crucially, on who paid the tax and national insurance bills that financed the total.

Fourthly, even if one generation is a "net gainer", this does not, as we shall see, necessarily mean that successive generations are "net losers". The analogy with an unsustainable chain letter game (Thomson 1991: 9) may be misleading. The usual kind of chain letter – with the numbers involved multiplying at each stage – is unsustainable: the first participants may each receive 64 postcards (or £64) from those further down the chain in return for the one they each sent, but the process cannot continue indefinitely without the world's entire population becoming involved, after which further participants become hard to find.

Seen from the perspective of the early 1990s, however, the welfare state, in Britain at least, no longer looks to be growing explosively. Rather, it seems – measured as a share of national income – to have grown rapidly in the thirty years after the Second World War, but to have stabilized since the mid-1970s (Hills 1993). There may, indeed, have been winners and losers as the welfare state has grown to maturity (if that is the correct way to describe it), but the approximate stability since the late 1970s is not so obviously unsustainable as to imply that currently young generations cannot get back something close to what they put in.

This brings up the final point. Since the welfare state does affect people "from cradle to grave", it may be misleading to look at just one part of their lives – even what seems quite a long period, like 30 years – and conclude that they have gained or lost. The calculation can be made only standing at the graveside, looking back over a period of up to a century.

This chapter sets out to explore whether there is evidence for intergenerational inequity – and the existence of a "welfare generation" – in Britain in the way in which the benefits from and costs of the major components of social spending (education, health and social security) have been distributed since the 1920s. It is, in effect, an exercise in "generational accounting" of the kind called for by Kotlikoff (1992), in his book of that title.

The next section discusses the issues involved in measuring intergenerational equity (or its absence). The third summarizes the empirical findings for the period up to 1991. The fourth explores the effects of extending the analysis with projections up to 2041. The data used and their sources are described in detail in the appendix to Hills (1992).[2]

What do we mean by "intergenerational equity"?

A large part of the operation of the welfare state consists of effective transfers between one stage and another in the same people's lives. At any given moment, a particular cohort may be receiving net benefits from or making net payments into the collective pool, but at other times the reverse may be the case. The problem is how to add together the net flows occurring at different times to give a "life-time total".

First, because of inflation, it is clearly incorrect to say that someone who "paid in" £1 in 1921 and "got back" £1 in 1991 has broken even in any meaningful sense. At the very least, we are interested in real, inflation-adjusted, amounts. Secondly, even measuring everything in real terms, a problem remains. The same amount of real purchasing power now is worth more than the same amount at some point in the future. We should therefore discount amounts received at different times by some real interest rate.

The approach used here is to say that payments in and out should be taken as balancing if they represent the same value – or sacrifice – in terms of contemporary living standards. If in one year, someone pays in the equivalent of 20 per cent of that year's average per capita income, then this would be balanced by a receipt in a later year equivalent to 20 per cent of the later year's average per capita income.

Receipts from and payments for the welfare state are measured here as percentages of contemporary GDP per capita. In 1991–2, GDP per capita in the UK was just over £10,000, while in 1921 it was just under £100. An age cohort that paid £1 million into the welfare state in 1921 thus would be taken as being treated neutrally if, for instance, it got about £100 million out in 1991.

This is equivalent to using the real rate of growth in per capita income as the real discount rate. This has the intuitive appeal that, measured in this way, a "steady state" welfare state would be "generationally neutral". That is, with successive cohorts of constant size, welfare spending taking a constant percentage of GDP, and no change in the ratios between spending on people of different ages, no generation would be a net gainer or a net loser. Each cohort would make the same tax and national insurance contributions to pay for welfare services and would receive services and benefits costing the same amount as each other, when measured in units of GDP per capita. Other implicit discount rates would imply that intergenerationally fair welfare states were either unsustainable (if the discount rate was higher than the real per capita growth rate), or were ever-diminishing (if the reverse was true). Neither alternative seems satisfactory.

What is a "generation"?

A second issue is the definition of what constitutes a "generation". On the one hand, the narrower the age range used the better, since even quite small differences in birth dates can, as a result of wars or the economic cycle, be associated with large differences in life-time circumstances (Johnson & Falkingham 1992: 6). On the other hand, we do not have the data to allocate spending and taxation by very narrow age ranges. The narrowest age bands for which the necessary information is available are five year age cohorts.

Table 3.1   Age cohorts used in the analysis.

Cohort	Born[a]	Age in 1991[b]	Representative	Size of cohort when 15–19 (million)	Size of cohort in 1991 (million)
1	1901–06	85–89	Alec Douglas-Home	3.98	0.62
2	1906–11	80–84	Barbara Castle	4.03	1.24
3	1911–16	75–79	Harold Wilson	3.87	1.81
4	1916–21	70–74	Denis Healey	3.55	2.22
5	1921–6	65–69	Margaret Thatcher	3.74	2.70
6	1926–31	60–64	Geoffrey Howe	3.28	2.81
7	1931–6	55–59	Michael Heseltine	3.07	2.85
8	1936–41	50–54	John Smith	3.21	3.01
9	1941–6	45–49	John Major	3.58	3.43
10	1946–51	40–44	Gordon Brown	4.15	4.04
11	1951–6	35–39	Tony Blair	3.70	3.68
12	1956–61	30–34	Charles Kennedy	4.01	4.10
13	1961–6	25–29	Matthew Taylor	4.47	4.62
14	1966–71	20–24	–	4.34	4.36
15	1971–6	15–19	–	3.56	3.59
16	1976–81	10–14	–	–	3.36
17	1981–6	5–9	–	–	3.53
18	1986–91	0–4	–	–	3.75

a. Years starting in April.
b. April 1991.

The cohorts used are described in Table 3.1. They are those in successive five year age groups at each census (i.e. in April), starting with
the cohort born between April 1901 and March 1906. This group –
"Cohort 1" – were aged between 85 and 89 in April 1991. In order to
put some flesh on the analysis, the table also lists a "representative"
for each of the cohorts born by 1966. In the case of Cohort 1 this is Sir
Alec Douglas-Home, the late Lord Home. If David Thomson's identification of a "welfare generation" born between 1920 and 1945 proved
correct for Britain, it would be Cohorts 5 to 9 – the "Thatcher to Major
generation" – who would be the net beneficiaries from the welfare
state.

The size of these cohorts varies, and this may affect their fortunes in
various ways. Larger cohorts may, for instance, face tougher labour
market conditions. As far as this analysis is concerned, one might
expect larger cohorts to gain from the way in which they can spread
out the financing cost of pensions and other provision for the elderly
when they are young, although this might be offset if smaller succes-

sor generations were only prepared to pay less generous pensions to them. For smaller cohorts, the reverse might be true (see Ermisch 1990: 46 for a discussion).

Table 3.1 shows the relative sizes of each cohort as it reached age 15–19, the largest being Cohort 13 born between 1961 and 1966 (the "Matthew Taylor" cohort), which was nearly 50 per cent larger than Cohort 7 (the "Heseltine" cohort) born between 1931 and 1936. Figure 3.1 shows how the sizes of the six cohorts used to illustrate the analysis have changed between 1911 and 1991. As well as demonstrating the variation in size between cohorts, it also shows that, even if one covers the whole period from 1911 to 1991, only the first cohort has got near to the end of its life. The others have many years of the welfare state to go (assuming that this survives in some form), years that have to be allowed for in some way if we are to make a meaningful comparison of life-time positions.

Incidence assumptions

It would be possible to allocate spending (and the taxes that finance it) on a year-by-year basis. To save computation, however, the approach here is to use spending – in units of GDP per capita – in every fifth year as representative of spending levels over a five year period.

Spending is allocated to those on whom it is directly spent and it is valued at the amount which it costs the public sector. Either assumption could be questioned. The true incidence of any benefit may not be on its direct beneficiaries. For instance, education spending is allocated to the children and young people at school or college. It may, however, be that the true beneficiaries of some of this spending are their parents, who would have paid for their children's education themselves, if the state had not. Or the beneficiaries might include a wide range of age cohorts, who gain from the higher level of economic performance resulting from better education and training (including the direct beneficiaries' children and parents); this is a form of the general "spillover" problem with incidence analysis. Similarly, in the absence of state pensions, working age children might have helped more to support their elderly parents, and so might really be the beneficiaries of part of pensions spending. However, such wider effects are not allowed for here.[3]

Secondly, the true value to its beneficiary of a service provided in kind like education or health care might be very different from the amount that it costs the state to provide. Inefficiencies or restricted choices might mean that recipients would put a lower value on services than their cost. Alternatively, the state might be providing – for instance, through the NHS – services that would have a far higher market value than their cost. We have no way of allowing for such differences between cost and value, so we are forced to use cost.

Looking at entire cohorts

The analysis looks at the position of age cohorts as a whole. Within each cohort some may do better, and others worse than the cohort average. Such intra-cohort variation and the factors that create it are explored in detail in Falkingham & Hills (1995), including an examination of the effects of the welfare state as it was structured in the mid-1980s on the members of a single (synthetic) cohort. Unfortunately, we do not have the longitudinal survey data to look at such variation within actual cohorts over the historical past. However, we can look at the average position of successive cohorts about which such variation takes place.

An alternative approach would be to look at the experience of "typical" members of each cohort and to work out how they would have been affected by the rules of the benefit and taxation systems at each stage in their lives. While this approach certainly generates some insights, it may be misleading if one cannot identify truly typical life-histories. Given the range of varying circumstances involved, to do this accurately one would need a huge range of different cases.

If one does not allow for variation in circumstances between cohorts, the results in terms of their receipts and tax payments may be misleading. For instance, Figure 3.1 shows that mortality patterns have changed: later cohorts live longer, which means they will collect pensions and benefit from health care over longer periods. Failing to allow for this will understate the relative gains from the pension system for later cohorts.

For that reason the aggregate approach used here seems preferable, giving insights of comparable value to other distributional analysis that looks at variations between groups split in one way (such as gender, education or income), abstracting from further variation caused by other factors.

Summary

What is reported below is a fairly standard, first round, incidence exercise looking at the distribution of the benefits of public spending

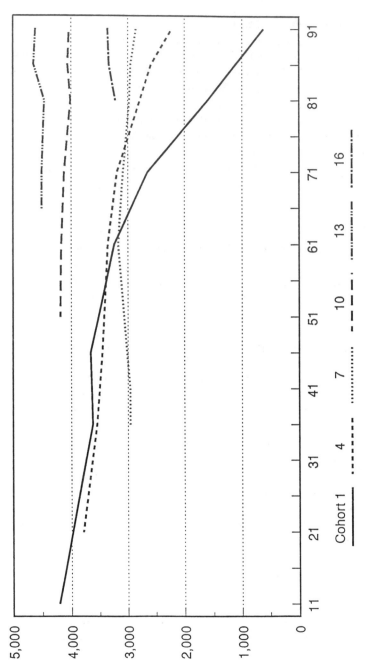

Figure 3.1 Size of cohort (Great Britain, 000s).

on education, health and social security, and the costs of the taxes that finance them. However, the allocation is not for a single year and between different income groups but is for a long time period and between successive five year age cohorts.

To be a "welfare generation", one of these cohorts would have to take out more than it puts in – that is, receive, over its completed lifetime, greater benefits than the taxes it pays to finance the welfare state, with amounts at different dates measured in relation to living standards (GDP per capita) at that point. For a generation that was "born to pay" – to quote Longman's (1987) title, describing those who will have to pay for US baby boomers in retirement – the reverse would be true.

Intergenerational distribution 1921 to 1991

The benefits people receive from the welfare state follow a marked life-cycle pattern. Education is concentrated early in life, while both health and social security spending are much higher after pension age than before it. By contrast, the taxes that finance welfare spending are much higher for the population of working age than for the young or old.

The result of this is that if one calculates the cumulative net receipts going, on average, to the survivors at each age in any given cohort, they follow a pronounced "wave pattern". This is shown for every third cohort in our exercise in Figure 3.2. For the earliest cohort, cumulative receipts up to age 90 can be shown; for Cohort 16, the picture extends only as far as age 15.

For each cohort, up to age 20, people are gaining, mainly through the education system. After that, their accumulated surplus first reduces and then turns into a deficit as average tax payments in people's working lives exceed average health and social security receipts. After retirement, tax payments drop, health and social security receipts rise steeply, and eventually the average cohort member surviving long enough goes into life-time surplus.

What the diagram shows is that with the increase in the scale of the welfare state in the 30 years after the Second World War, the amplitude of this wave has increased. The cumulative net benefits by age 20 are higher for each successive cohort, but so is the accumulated net deficit by age 60.

65

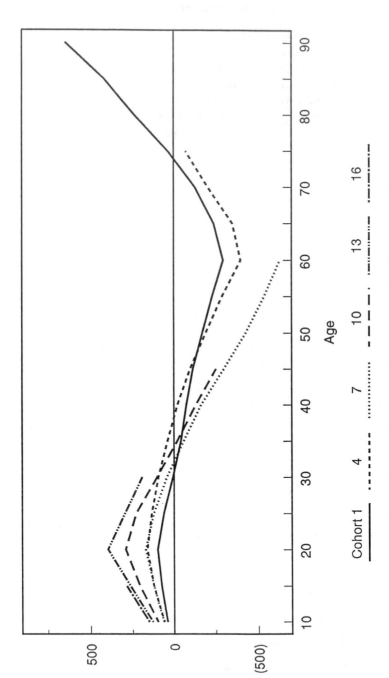

Figure 3.2 Cumulative net gain per survivor (% of GDP per capita).

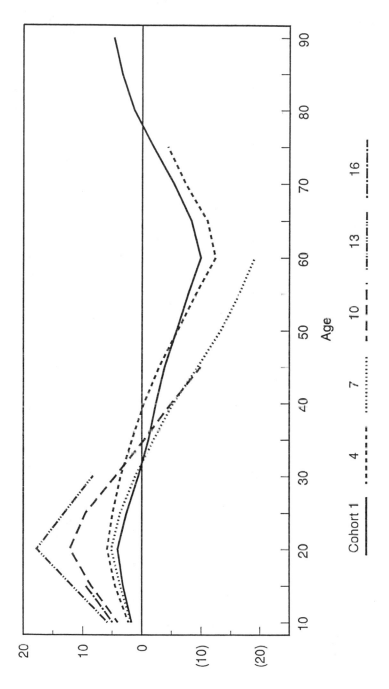

Figure 3.3 Cumulative net gain for cohort (millions of GDP per capita).

What the diagram does *not* give us, however, is an answer to the main question under investigation of equity between cohorts. This is first because later cohorts are surviving longer than earlier ones – so the average member may survive long enough to be in a better life-time position than the average member of an earlier cohort, even if the position at any given age is worse. Secondly, only Cohort 1 has got near to the end of its life. Using data up to 1991, it is not at all clear how later cohorts will end up. Things look bad for Cohort 7, down by the equivalent of more than six years' worth of average income for each survivor aged 60, well below Cohorts 1 and 4 at the same age. But more generous pensions and better funded health care throughout retirement might yet change the end result.

Figure 3.3 shows the cumulative net position of each cohort as a whole, built up from the receipts of those surviving to each age, thus allowing for differential survival rates. In this diagram, a "welfare generation" would end up above the break-even line; those "born to

Table 3.2 Cumulative net receipts by cohort in 1991 (millions of GDP per capita).

Cohort	Age in 1991	Education	Health (low variation)	Social security	Taxes[a]	Net benefit[b]
1	85–9	3.8	8.2	21.6	−28.8	+4.8
2	80–84	3.9	8.8	22.6	−32.8	+2.7
3	75–9	4.2	8.4	21.0	−33.8	−0.2
4	70–74	4.8	6.8	17.6	−33.7	−4.4
5	65–9	5.2	7.0	14.6	−38.8	−12.1
6	60–64	4.6	5.7	9.5	−37.4	−17.6
7	55–9	4.6	5.0	7.3	−36.0	−19.1
8	50–54	6.7	4.7	6.8	−34.1	−15.9
9	45–9	9.6	4.7	7.0	−34.1	−12.7
10	40–44	12.0	5.3	7.5	−34.6	−9.9
11	35–9	12.1	4.2	7.2	−25.9	−2.4
12	30–34	14.7	4.3	6.4	−21.6	+3.9
13	25–9	15.3	4.5	4.6	−16.0	+8.3
14	20–24	14.3	3.9	2.5	−7.6	+13.1
15	15–19	12.0	3.0	0.5	—	+15.6
16	10–14	7.1	2.5	—	—	+9.5
17	5–9	3.4	2.2	—	—	+5.5
18	0–4	—	2.1	—	—	+2.1

a. Taxes required to finance welfare services only.
b. Hills (1995) describes the way in which these results are built up for the separate services – education, health, and social security – and for the taxes which finance them.

pay" would end up below it. Table 3.2 gives more detailed figures for the cumulative positions by 1991 of each of the 18 cohorts born between 1901 and 1991.

At this point in the analysis, only one thing is clear: Cohorts 1 and 2 – the Alec Douglas-Home and Barbara Castle cohorts – do appear as net winners. By 1991, these groups' cumulative net receipts from the welfare state had already exceeded their net payments into it. Cohort 3 – the Harold Wilson cohort – had also almost reached break-even by the time its members had reached 80, so it too should end up as a net gainer. Beyond this, it is hard to say anything with certainty. Looking at Figure 3.3, Cohort 4 (Denis Healey's), tracking just below Cohort 1, looks as if it too will end up as a net gainer, but for later ones it is hard to tell.

This leads to one firm conclusion: it is very hard to say anything definitive about intergenerational equity on the basis of incomplete life-histories. Unless we project the analysis forward into the future, there is little we can say about cohorts born since the 1920s.

Projections of receipts and payments to 2041

While the future – particularly over the 50 year period that we need to examine – is clearly highly uncertain, we do have some information to work on. First, we have official projections of the numbers of each cohort surviving to a given age (in this case, those in OPCS 1993). Secondly, we have the Government Actuary's (1990) projections of the future costs of the State Earnings-Related Pension Scheme (SERPS), which represents the largest change to the future shape of the welfare state about which we already know. Beyond this, we can work only on the basis of current spending patterns.

The base projection

The base projection here uses spending patterns as they were in relation to average incomes in 1991–2 for each group of a given age, and assumes that groups of the same age benefit from the equivalent level of spending in the future. Thus, 10–14 year olds were benefiting from annual education spending equivalent to 24 per cent of GDP per capita in 1991–2 (about £2,400), so it is assumed that 10–14 year olds will continue to benefit from the same level of spending per head relative to average incomes in the future.

The exception to this is that projected SERPS receipts are used rather than those actually being received by particular age groups in 1991–2, and the changing build-up of receipts for different cohorts is allowed for. The net benefits included from greater SERPS receipts are lower than the gross benefits to allow for the increased tax payments and reduced means-tested benefits that will result from them.[4]

The first column of Table 3.3 shows the projected total of spending on education, health and social security as a percentage of GDP that results from this process. Thus, if spending on the three services for people of a given age continued to have the same value in relation to average incomes as it did in 1991, their cost would rise from 22.2 per cent of GDP in 1991 to 26.3 per cent in 2041. This 4.1 percentage point increase in the share of national income needed to finance the welfare state over a 50 year period contrasts with a 16.6 percentage point increase over the previous 50 years. The bulk of the increase comes from demographic factors – the ageing population.

This increased cost of the three services is assumed to be met by greater tax and national insurance payments by all age groups, with the relativities between individuals of each age staying as they were in 1991.

Table 3.3 Projected total spending on education, health and social security 1991 to 2041 (% of GDP, GB).

	1991 spending patterns[a]	Social security price-linked[b]	Health spending rises by 0.5% per annum above GDP per capita[c]
1991	22.2	22.2	22.2
1996	22.3	21.4	22.5
2001	22.6	20.9	23.0
2006	22.9	20.6	23.5
2011	23.5	20.3	24.3
2016	24.0	20.1	25.1
2021	24.5	19.8	25.8
2026	25.2	19.7	26.9
2031	25.9	19.6	27.9
2036	26.3	19.3	28.7
2041	26.3	18.8	29.1

a. Allowing for build-up of net receipts from SERPS (on earnings-linked basis).

b. Allowing for net receipts from SERPS (on price-linked basis).

c. And using high variation of health by age.

Results from the base projection

Figures 3.4 and 3.5 and Table 3.4 give the results of using projections on this basis. From Figure 3.4 it can be seen that, at any given age from 30, the position of surviving members of Cohort 7 is worse than that of those from any of the other cohorts. For later cohorts, the relative decline in position is reversed, although the later cohorts do not end up in as favourable a position as Cohorts 1 and 4.

However, later cohorts are surviving longer. The population projections used suggest a median life-span of 73 for Cohort 1, 77 for Cohort 4, 81 for Cohort 7 and 83 for Cohort 10. In each case, these ages are remarkably close to the break-even point at which cumulative net benefits become positive.

Figure 3.5 shows results for cohorts as a whole up to age 95 (beyond which there are too few survivors to make any appreciable difference). Cohorts 1 and 4 end up as net gainers, Cohort 7 breaks even, but Cohort 10 ends up as net gainers, longer life expectancy having a noticeable effect after age 80. Even projecting forward to 2041 is not

Table 3.4 Cumulative net receipts by cohort in 2041 (1991 spending pattern maintained, millions of GDP per capita).

Cohort	Age in 2041	Education	Health (low variation)	Social security	Taxes[a]	Net benefit
1	–	3.8	8.7	22.2	−29.2	5.5
2	–	3.9	10.4	24.6	−33.8	5.2
3	–	4.2	11.3	25.5	−36.0	5.0
4	–	4.8	11.5	25.6	−37.6	4.4
5	–	5.2	13.1	27.6	−45.1	0.8
6	–	4.6	12.9	28.1	−45.8	−0.2
7	–	4.6	12.9	29.7	−46.7	0.5
8		6.7	13.9	32.7	−51.0	2.4
9	–	9.6	16.2	38.6	−59.8	4.6
10	90–94	12.0	19.5	45.7	−72.3	4.9
11	85–9	12.1	16.2	41.2	−65.9	3.6
12	80–84	14.7	16.0	43.0	−72.5	1.3
13	75–9	15.3	16.1	43.0	−79.9	−5.5
14	70–74	14.8	13.0	35.2	−74.6	−11.6
15	65–9	13.4	10.0	24.2	−61.5	−14.0
16	60–64	12.7	8.2	16.7	−56.6	−19.0
17	55–9	13.7	8.0	13.6	−57.4	−22.1
18	50–54	14.6	7.9	12.1	−53.5	−19.0

a. Taxes required to finance welfare services only. Tax receipts resulting from rise in SERPS netted out of social security.

71

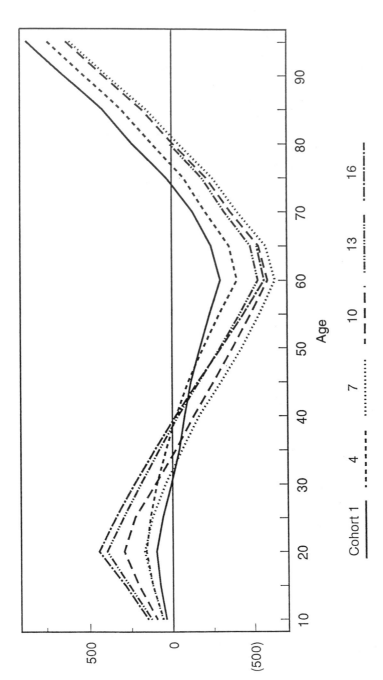

Figure 3.4 Projected cumulative net gain per survivor (1991 spending patterns, % of GDP per capita).

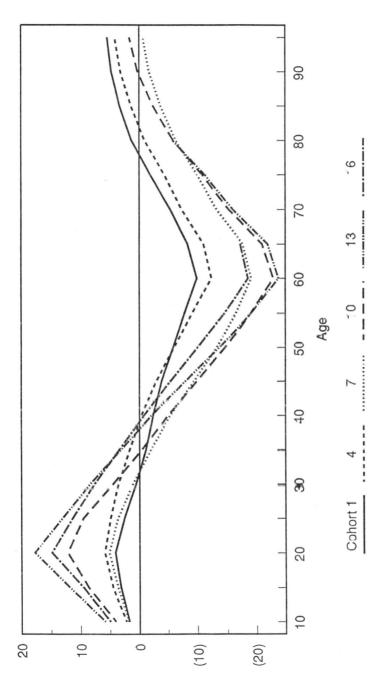

Figure 3.5 Projected cumulative net gain for cohort (1991 spending patterns, millions of GDP per capita).

long enough to give a definitive result for Cohorts 13 and 16, but they too look as if they will end up narrowly as net gainers.

Perhaps the most striking feature of the diagram, however, is the closeness of the end-positions to break-even. By and large, each cohort gets out something close to what it puts in. In contrast to the statements about "considerable injustices between different generations" and about the unsustainability of the welfare state quoted at the start of this chapter, the British welfare state comes out of this analysis as remarkably well balanced.

Table 3.4 shows more detailed results for all of the cohorts born between 1901 and 1991. The first four cohorts – Douglas-Home to Healey – are net gainers. The next three (Thatcher to Heseltine) make small net losses or gains. After that, Cohorts 8 to 12 (Smith to Kennedy) end up as net gainers, and it looks as if Cohort 13 (Taylor) will do so too.

On this base projection, therefore, the conclusion is very different from that described by Thomson for New Zealand. The only apparent loser – and then only narrowly – is the cohort born between 1926 and 1931. The clearest "welfare generation" is those born between 1901 and 1921.

Those born between 1921 and 1936 do not do so well. This partly reflects the time path of the expansion of the welfare state. Cohorts 6 and 7 are also two of the smallest cohorts. This gives some support to the idea that smaller cohorts lose out from having few members among whom to spread the costs of paying for welfare when they are of working age.

Table 3.5 shows the same results recalculated to express the position of the cohort as a whole as an average per member of the cohort alive at age 15–19. It shows how life-time gross receipts per member build up from the equivalent of just under nine years' worth of GDP per capita for the earliest cohort to over eighteen for Cohort 10. Tax payments to finance the welfare state also grow towards the same level, but the growth comes a little later (and from a slightly lower base). The result of this is that the earliest cohorts – gaining from the rise in receipts but not affected so much by the rise in tax – end up as net gainers, to the extent of an average of something over one year's worth of GDP per capita for each member.

However, the scale of these net gains and losses is not enormous. The final column of the table shows the receipts of each cohort as a percentage of the tax it pays. Apart from the first four, the receipts of each of the cohorts with complete projected life-times is within 8 per

Table 3.5 Projected life-time receipts and tax payments until 2041 (1991 spending pattern maintained).[a]

Cohort	Born	Age in 1991	Size of cohort when 15–19 (million)	Cumulative receipts and payments (GDP per capita per member at 15–19)			
				Receipts	Tax	Net gain	Receipts as % tax
1	1901–06	85–9	4.0	8.7	7.3	1.4	119
2	1906–11	80–84	4.0	9.7	8.4	1.3	115
3	1911–16	75–9	3.9	10.6	9.3	1.3	114
4	1916–21	70–74	3.6	11.8	10.6	1.2	112
5	1921–6	65–9	3.7	12.3	12.1	0.2	102
6	1926–31	60–64	3.2	13.9	14.0	–0.1	100
7	1931–6	55–9	3.1	15.4	15.2	0.2	101
8	1936–41	50–54	3.2	16.6	15.9	0.7	105
9	1941–6	45–9	3.6	18.0	16.7	1.3	108
10	1946–51	40–44	4.1	18.6	17.4	1.2	107
Incomplete life-times							
11(to 90)	1951–6	35–9	3.7	18.8	17.8	1.0	105
12 (to 85)	1956–61	30–34	4.0	18.4	18.1	0.3	102
13 (to 80)	1961–6	25–9	4.5	16.7	17.9	–1.2[b]	93

a. But allowing for build-up of net receipts from SERPS (on earnings-linked basis). Health on low variation basis.
b. Cohort 13 is in a slightly less favourable position at age 80 than was Cohort 10 at the same age.

cent of the tax that it pays. Even the first four cohorts "pay for" between 80 and 90 per cent of the benefits that they receive. Again, this is a long way from being generations that "make contributions which cover only a fraction of their benefits".

To summarize, what appears to have happened in Britain is the following. During the twentieth century, public spending on education, health and social security has grown from a low level to around 22 per cent of national income. If levels of provision for any age were to remain unchanged relative to average incomes (apart from SERPS), their total cost would grow to just over 26 per cent of national income over the next 50 years.[5] This spending is financed mainly by the working population at any time. Because the benefits of the welfare state are – for obvious reasons – weighted towards the latter parts of people's lives, there is a generation born in the early years of the century that has benefited from the expansion in the welfare state in their own retirement, but whose life-time tax payments reflected the somewhat smaller levels of provision for their parents' generation. Later generations tend roughly to break even.

Alternative assumptions about the future

All of this is based on the idea that the welfare state has reached some kind of maturity, and that relative levels of provision will now remain constant for any given age group. This is not, of course, necessarily so. First, current government policy is not to link social security benefits to current living standards as the base projection assumes, but to link them to prices. Benefits will thus gradually lose value in terms of average incomes and the accounting unit – GDP per capita – used here. The second column of Table 3.3 shows the effect on the overall total of government spending if this policy was followed for the next 50 years (assuming annual real per capita growth of 1.5 per cent, in line with the assumption made by the Government Actuary, 1990). In this case, the cost of the three services falls from 22 per cent of GDP in 1991 to 19 per cent in 2041.

Alternatively, there may be pressures for the welfare state to grow. For instance, spending on health care for given age groups has risen more rapidly than average incomes for much of the period since the Second World War (and when it did not in the early 1980s, the strains were apparent). In addition, the results presented above are sensitive to the assumptions made about health spending by age. Allowing for greater variation by age would imply faster growth in spending as the population ages. The third column of Table 3.3 therefore shows the effects of adding an annual 0.5 per cent rise in the cost of health care (say, because of medical advance) to the base projection, and of assuming "high variation" in health spending with age.[6] In this case, the total cost of welfare spending reaches more than 29 per cent of GDP by 2041.

These alternatives represent significantly different paths for the welfare state: in the first, it is rolled back from its current importance, while in the second it resumes its growth. As a test of the sensitivity of the base results, Table 3.6 shows the effects of using these alternative projections on the position of the cohorts born up to 1966.

The first part of the table shows the effects of price-linking social security. As far as the four earliest cohorts are concerned, there is little effect by comparison with the base projection: the 1.5 per cent per year relative decline in the value of social security payments makes little difference until after most of their members have died. However, the

Table 3.6 Projected life-time receipts and tax payments until 2041 (variations to 1991 spending pattern).

Cohort	Social security price-linked[a] Cumulative receipts and payments (GDP per capita per member at age 15–19)			Receipt as % tax	Health spending rises 0.5% per annum above GDP per capita[b] Cumulative receipts and payments (GDP per capita per member at age 15–19)			Receipt as % tax
	Receipts	Tax	Net		Receipts	Tax	Net	
1	8.7	7.3	1.4	119	9.1	7.3	1.7	124
2	9.6	8.4	1.2	115	10.1	8.4	1.7	120
3	10.5	9.2	1.2	113	11.1	9.3	1.8	119
4	11.5	10.5	1.0	110	12.4	10.6	1.8	117
5	11.7	11.9	−0.2	98	12.9	12.1	0.8	107
6	13.0	13.7	−0.7	95	14.7	14.0	0.7	105
7	14.0	14.8	−0.8	94	16.3	15.3	1.0	107
8	14.8	15.3	−0.5	97	17.7	16.1	1.6	110
9	15.6	15.9	−0.2	99	19.2	17.0	2.3	113
10	15.8	16.3	−0.5	97	19.9	17.8	2.2	112
Incomplete life-times								
11 (to 90)	15.8	16.4	−0.6	96	19.8	18.2	1.6	109
12 (to 85)	15.2	16.3	−1.1	93	19.1	18.6	0.5	103
13 (to 80)	13.5	15.8	−2.2	86	17.2	18.5	−1.3	93

a. Assumed to fall by 1.5% in relation to GDP pc. Allows for price-linked SERPS.
b. With "high variation" in health receipts with age.

change pushes cohorts from Cohort 5 (the Thatcher cohort) onwards into making net losses, although they still receive back over 90 per cent of the tax they pay.

As the welfare state scaled down in this way those currently in middle age would receive significantly lower pensions themselves in 30 or so years' time, but would not save very much in tax from only slightly reduced pensions paid to their parents' generation. If they wanted to maintain their relative living standards in retirement, they would have to pay more privately towards their own pensions at the same time as paying the tax bill for those currently retired. Eventually, for much later cohorts, social security (apart, as it happens, from SERPS, which is in certain ways linked to earnings) would cease to have very much importance either way and the system would return to some kind of lower level intergenerational balance. In short, the current price-linking policy is of most disadvantage to those cohorts who are currently middle aged.

As one might expect, Table 3.6 shows that the alternative scenario of a gradual build-up of health costs while the relative values of other items remained the same would have the reverse effect. The gains of the first few cohorts are increased by comparison with the base case because the "high variation" assumption about health spending allocates more of the spending in the 1980s and 1990s to them. The position of subsequent cohorts is also improved, although none of them reaches as favourable a position as the first four.

This analysis rests on particular ways of allocating the benefits from and costs of the welfare state between different age groups. Some of these might be done in alternative ways, and it might be that the conclusions reached would then be different. However, Hills (1995) presents a sensitivity analysis showing the receipts of each cohort as a percentage of the taxes they pay under seven variations by comparison with the base case. While that analysis shows that the use of different assumptions can affect the precise position of any of the cohorts, none of the combinations suggests the presence of a cohort that only pays for a "fraction of its benefits", or that only receives back a fraction of the taxes it pays. While there may be "welfare generations" to the extent of receiving net gains of up to 25 per cent of the tax they pay, the greatest net loss for those with completed lives by 2041 does not exceed 6 per cent of the taxes they pay under any of the scenarios. It is hard to identify a generation that is "born to pay" to any great extent.

Conclusion

First, it does appear that those born between 1901 and 1921 will end up getting rather more out of the welfare state than they put in, although even this generation will have "paid for" between 80 per cent and 90 per cent of what they get out under most assumptions. Of course, as for other cohorts, individual members may fare far better or far worse than this average.

Secondly, it is not possible to reach conclusions about later cohorts unless one makes some kind of projection of what will happen to them in the future. If one assumes that education, health and social security will (with the exception of allowing for the build-up of receipts from SERPS) maintain their current values in relation to contemporary living standards over the next 50 years, cohorts born

CONCLUSION

between 1921 and 1966 will end up roughly breaking even, generally making small gains. This picture would be little changed if, on top of the effects of demographic change, health spending for people of a given age grew somewhat faster than average incomes.

However, if social security payments continued to be price- rather than income-linked over the next 50 years, the picture would deteriorate for those born after 1921, and all the subsequent cohorts examined would end up as net losers, albeit narrowly (they still get back more than 90 per cent of what they would have "put in").

Alternative ways of allocating education and health benefits and of allocating the tax required to finance spending also increase or decrease the estimated net gains or losses for particular cohorts, but they do not affect the overall conclusion – that for most cohorts aggregate life-time benefits are not very different from aggregate life-time taxes, and it is hard to identify a "born to pay" generation that gets back significantly less than it puts in.

Earlier in the chapter it was suggested that the analogy of an explosive – and unstable – "chain letter" game was misleading as a description of the operation of the British welfare state. A better analogy might be the following. A single line of people – stretching indefinitely into the distance – sit next to one another on chairs. Each has a box of chocolates. When the game starts, each in turn passes their box of chocolates to the person on the left. The person at the left-hand end of the line ends up a net gainer, with two boxes of chocolates. Every one else eventually breaks even, ending up with a single box of chocolates, provided that the line carries on indefinitely and that no-one changes the rules. However, if someone somewhere down the line were to panic in the interval between passing on their original box and receiving their neighbour's, and say that the game ought to be stopped, it is they who would end up as the only losers.

In the case of the British welfare state, those born in the early years of the century are the equivalent of the person at the left-hand end of the line, and they end up as clear net gainers. Given that they lived through the Depression of the 1930s and were the generation who had to fight the Second World War, it might be thought churlish to begrudge them this gain; after all, intergenerational equity is not just about the welfare state.

Those of us born later are the equivalent of those further down the line. In the end we shall generally get back what we put in – provided that we do not start calling the game off by abolishing or substantially

79

scaling down the welfare state. However, individual members of a particular cohort may well have very different interests from its average member. Date of birth is only one of the many characteristics determining how the welfare state affects people. For individuals, the differences in the net life-time effects of the welfare state that result from their income levels, gender, and family circumstances may be much more important.

Notes

1. This chapter contains an edited version of material also contained in Hills (1995) to which the reader is referred for more detailed discussion. Full details of the data used can be found in Hills (1992). The author is very grateful to David Thomson for comments on an earlier version and to participants in the 1992 British Association annual conference, and in seminars at the London School of Economics and University of Sussex for helpful suggestions.
2. The data used are updated in three respects from the sources described in Hills (1992). First, spending figures for 1991–2 are based on the revised out-turn estimates given in HM Treasury (1993), Table 2.5, and associated departmental reports. Secondly, GDP per capita is based on revised GDP figures for 1991–2 (ibid., Table 2.1). Thirdly, the population projections used are those published in Office of Population Censuses and Surveys (1993), using a 1991 base, rather than the 1985 base used in the earlier exercise. None of these revisions makes a substantial difference to the overall conclusions.
3. In Hills (1995) we test the sensitivity of the results to this by examining the effect of allocating education to parents rather than their children.
4. The results do not allow for the increase in women's pension age to 65 after 2010.
5. Of course, the economic cycle and changing levels of unemployment may be superimposed on – and at times be larger than – these purely demographic and structural effects. In effect, the projections assume age-related unemployment patterns following those of 1991–2.
6. The rationale behind the alternative ways of allocating health spending by age is discussed in Hills (1992).

CHAPTER 4

Ties that bind

Dorothy Jerrome

Relationship is the worst ship that ever bloody well sailed. (Wife of police sergeant, aged 58, Christmas 1984, Mass Observation Archive)

Introduction

This chapter examines the strength of family ties, particularly across the generations. It covers the range and content of contemporary relationships, paying particular attention to parents and children in the second half of life, and grandparents and grandchildren, and siblings. The focus of my interest is British society. I have drawn on the literature of social gerontology and material from the British Mass Observation Archive based at the University of Sussex. This unique collection of autobiographical writing casts new light on the experience of "family", reminding us of the need for flexibility in theorizing about this domain (Jerrome 1994a).

As the opening quotation suggests, relationships are not always positive, though it is difficult to know how to interpret the sentiments expressed here. How does one measure the strength of family ties? What facts or feelings should be regarded as significant? Links between generations of family members take many forms. No single concept describes their variety and complexity, though there are three that, spanning the disciplines of history, sociology and psychology, help to focus our attention. They are continuity, solidarity and generativity. We might ask about the link between historical *continuity* (the family as a system continuing over time), intergenerational *solidarity* (measured in terms of interaction, attitudes and feelings) and *generativity* (a psychological concept referring to an adult's need to perpetuate him- or herself through influencing the next generation).

In this chapter some of these concerns are explored. The chapter starts with a discussion of the concept of family solidarity and ways of measuring it. A range of dimensions is offered that provide a framework for the analysis of intergenerational ties. The next section concentrates on contact between family members. It is followed by a discussion of feelings, for which the concept of attachment provides a starting point. Special attention is given to grandparenthood as a key relationship. The discussion moves on to another dimension of solidarity – consensus, or the extent to which attitudes and values are shared. One set of attitudes in particular, concerning the family itself, is given detailed consideration. Finally, the discussion returns to the issue of conflict and consensus across the generations, sometimes experienced as "family" versus personal interest. In conclusion, some speculations are offered concerning the shape of the family in the future.

Family connectedness: dimensions of solidarity

There are some common beliefs about relationships between the generations. One is that they have weakened since the 1950s, mainly to the disadvantage of the older members; families are geographically dispersed and generally less committed to keeping in touch. A second belief is in what has become known as "the generation gap", the existence of conflict between the generations. A third notion is that exchanges between family members benefit older people rather than younger; they receive more help than they provide.

Academic concerns have mirrored these popular ideas. Research and writing on intergenerational relationships has taken a discernible path since the 1950s (Hagestad 1987). In the 1950s and 1960s the focus was the supposed isolation of the nuclear family. In the years after the student troubles of the 1960s attention shifted to the extent of similarity and difference between the generations, particularly in terms of attitudes. In the late 1970s and 1980s the emphasis shifted again, to patterns of help-giving and dependence between the old and their adult children. This was in recognition of demographic shifts and their negative impact on family life.

In the 1990s academic interest in relationships between the generations is broader and less problem-oriented than in those earlier decades. It still tends to focus on the parent–child relationship, that vertical link that provides continuity in the family system over time, but recognizes its capacity to cover most of the life-span.

Current thinking about the family as it develops over the decades goes beyond the issue of help-giving and receiving as a measure of the existence of bonds. Several measures are used. Contact and shared activities, attitudes and expectations, and feelings are all involved in family relationships. Space does not permit detailed discussions of all these dimensions of solidarity, which exist elsewhere (e.g. Acock 1984, Troll & Stapley 1985, Glass et al. 1986, Troll 1986, Bengston 1987, Hagestad 1987, Treas & Bengston 1987, Walker et al. 1987). I shall concentrate here on patterns of contact, the sense of closeness, similarity in ideas, and expectations about family life.

Patterns of contact

Family members keep in touch through visits, phone calls and letters. They share activities ranging from the informal (recreation, conversation, talking about important matters), through ceremonial or family ritual activities (gatherings, reunions, anniversaries) to the exchange of assistance.

We know that adult children see their parents often but the research tends to suffer from asymmetry. Older parents are asked if they are in contact with an adult child and one child is enough. But as Hagestad (1987) points out, we cannot assume that because most older parents have frequent contact with a middle-aged child, most middle-aged children have regular contact with elderly parents. We do not know the conditions under which there is great distance and little contact between adults and their parents: whether, apart from the one child who is in contact, there are others who have lost touch. It would be interesting to know under what circumstances adult children disappear, losing touch even with siblings. Material in the Mass Observation Archive indicates that this is not uncommon. Sometimes a gap is closed after many years. Contact is made after assiduous searching, only to find that the lost sheep would rather not get involved in family life (Jerrome 1994a).

"Family work" – the work of keeping in touch, providing services, keeping up with individual developments and disseminating family information – tends to be undertaken by women. Variously described as the linchpins of family contact, the family monitors, kinkeepers, it is they who orchestrate family get-togethers, keep track of birthdays and anniversaries, buy the presents, send the cards and make the phone calls. This appears to be the case in families with school-aged children and older families alike.

Ties are maintained by women, though sometimes under protest: "My husband's mother writes to me, and expects me to reply on behalf of my husband! I accept it now and carry on as I don't want to disappoint my mother-in-law. My husband never writes; his father has never written either!" A male Mass Observation writer expresses the general view that women will keep in touch with both sets of relatives. Indeed, there is astonishment and a sense of disbelief in his account of social situations where "when you ask how the relations are she only mentions hers, as if his didn't exist!" There is clearly no expectation that the husband might speak for himself, or the wife feel responsible for her relatives alone.

Hagestad quotes a study in which adults were asked to identify the adult child to whom they gave the most comfort, and the child from whom they received the most comfort. The diversity of parent–child relations increased with family size. However, the "loved one" and "the loving" children tended to be daughters who lived geographically close. Married daughters tend to have closer ties to parents than do married sons. This is particularly true for widowed mothers who see daughters as providers of emotional closeness and sons as more task-orientated and less frequent supporters.

The apparent weighting towards women in the performance of kinship roles might be a product of enquiry into processes that are typically female; in short, that it is an artefact of the research method. An emphasis on other exchanges – the payment of bills, for instance – might redress the balance (Margaret Forster's novel, *Have the men had enough?*, illustrates the gendered nature of family work along these lines). However, it is worth nothing that, in common with other studies of family involvement, the Mass Observation material on family life is overwhelmingly feminine. Of the 472 respondents who chose to write about the topic, 359 were women.

Sex is one of the four factors that appear to affect the nature of intergenerational contact. Marital status is the second. Unmarried offspring appear to maintain closer ties to ageing parents than do married children, at least in terms of being more likely to share housing with them. Among young adult daughters the difference is marked. The relationships of young married daughters with their middle-aged mothers are less interdependent than those of young single women and their mothers though ironically the mothers perceived their married daughters as being "more selfless" (Walker et al. 1987).

The third characteristic affecting contact is social class. As social class rises, nuclear families in a kinship network maintain greater distance between themselves. Older parents are less intensively involved with their adult children on a day-to-day basis, and socialization is expected to occur with peers rather than children. All this could be a consequence of geographical mobility. It might also reflect life-long expectations of friendship outside marriage, which have been linked to social class (Gavron 1966, O'Connor 1992).

Finally, patterns of contact vary between ethnic groups. However, the evidence is conflicting. While some American studies have found higher rates of contact between older blacks and their offspring, others have found that older whites tended to see their children and grandchildren more frequently. It is possible that outward migration of young blacks looking for jobs has an adverse effect on contact with elderly people, particularly in black working class families.

The British evidence, based on studies of inner city areas in Birmingham and Bristol, indicates differences between Asian and West Indian families in the degrees of contact and co-residence. There is evidence that proportionately more West Indian women live with younger people than their older white counterparts, at least in inner city areas. The pattern is even more pronounced in Asian households (Blakemore 1983) though the desire for closer contact is likely to be frustrated by inadequate space (Glendenning 1983). Clearly it is important to disregard stereotyped views of black family structure as invariably extended and highly interactive.

In one of the best known studies of intergenerational contact, by Bengston and associates, both generations reported relatively high levels of all types of activities, but there was one specific difference in perception. When estimating the amount of help given by the middle-aged child, the child concerned reported a higher level than did the parent. The parents reported giving less help to the children than the latter reported receiving. The parents thus tended to play down the practical exchanges between generations. They tended to emphasize the quality of affection and emotional closeness between the generations.

Family feeling: the affective dimension

Attachment is a concept usually used in relation to the early years of parenthood. It refers to dependence on a specific person for emotional support and includes the dislike and discomfort of being separated from that person (Walker et al. 1987). Life-span attachment theory, which since the mid-1980s has emerged in recognition of the life-long attachment between parents and children, builds on theories of bonding in childhood (Cicirelli 1983).

Despite the continuity of experience, parent–child relationships at each end of the life-span are dealt with separately, even to the extent that different terms are used (Hagestad 1987). Thus "parent–child relationships" invariably refers to the early years of parenting, with chronologically young children. The literature tends to refer to older parents and children in terms of "intergenerational relationships" and "older families", as if 90-year-old parents and 70-year-old children are inconceivable. In fact, life overlaps of this order are increasingly common (Hagestad 1985, Timaeus 1986, Gibson 1990) as families age together.

However, concentrating on the Omega phase of parent–child relationships, to use Hagestad's term, some conclusions may be drawn. It is evident that most adult children maintain some level of attachment behaviour (such as the wish to maintain in contact) in relation to elderly parents and that the relationship is an ongoing and viable one. Only a very few elderly people have lost contact with their adult children (Cicirelli 1983). In Cicirelli's own study, 87 per cent of adult children felt "close" or "very close" to their elderly mothers; very few felt "not close at all". Daughters felt closer than sons. There was a positive relationship between social class and feelings of closeness. This finding is confirmed by a study in which better overall relationships occurred in mothers and daughters whose life circumstances were better (Troll & Stapley 1985). Troll and Stapley also found that the relationship of mother and daughter is marked by discontinuity, with women's feelings of friendliness towards their mothers fluctuating somewhat over adulthood. However, very young women lacked empathy with both mothers and grandmothers. They seemed curiously unrelated to their woes or anything else. Perhaps they were preoccupied with the pursuit of partners or care of children, and had little familial concern left over. More importantly, the existence of generations above perhaps acted as a buffer against the concerns – of mortality, of physical decline – that might distress the middle generation.

The youngest generation of men in Troll and Stapley's three-generation study responded to family trouble by turning away from thoughts of older family members. On the other hand, their references to them were associated with much feeling, both positive and negative.

Children gain a great deal of satisfaction from their relationships with parents and report getting on well with them. A Mass Observer reports:

> My relationship with my mother changes as I get older (I am 35). I find I can speak my mind much more easily now and I would say that as well as being parents and daughter, we are also friends. They are the sort of people I would want to know even if we were not actually related.

However, in Cicirelli's study adult children were less likely to share intimate details of their lives and important decisions with their parents. (Parents know very little, for instance, about the state of their children's marriages. Those whose children divorce are sometimes taken by surprise: Troll 1986.) Presumably members of the peer group were chosen for this purpose.

In terms of conflict, very few children reported frequent conflict with their parents, while over one-third reported no conflict at all. Conflict centred mostly on one party's criticism of or intrusion into the other's habits or activities. However, they did expect an increase in conflict if they were to live together. It may be that most parents and adult children are able to minimize conflict by limiting the scope of the relationship. In extreme cases an unhappy *modus vivendi* is reached which amounts to estrangement (Jerrome 1994b).

Cicirelli's study investigated motives for interaction between parents and children to determine how far it rested on attachment or a sense of duty. He concluded that the adult child makes contact with the parent at least partly out of love and because the child wants to.

Despite these findings, the picture of family feeling is not altogether clear. Warmth in relationships is not easy to measure. In a longitudinal study of father–child relationships in later life, the researchers decided not even to speak of "closeness", since there was such a lack of consensus regarding its meaning (Hagestad 1987). For these fathers, all over 45, terms like "love", "caring" and "affection" were uncomfortable and difficult to discuss.

However, even in studies with relatively crude measures, two findings in particular are consistent: parents will describe the relationship more positively than the child, and reported closeness shows distinct sex differences. Parents are less likely to report negative changes in the relationship, while younger generations more readily report strain and conflict. Daughters appear to feel more closeness than sons, and are more likely to be named as the favourite children. The attachment of mothers and daughters across the generations is not affected by changes of role (Walker et al. 1987).

The asymmetry of attachment relationships is interesting. Why should parents consistently describe the relationship as better than their children do? An obvious explanation is that they have invested more in it, have more to lose if it fails and less time to rectify matters. Parents strive for continuity, while their children need change. The needs of older people for social continuity in the face of personal change and decline has been discussed elsewhere (Coleman & McCulloch 1985, Fiske & Chiriboga 1985). We can see how it might work in the context of the family by referring to Bengston's work on change and persistence in values and attitudes over the generations. He gives clearly the impression that parents have a need to minimize the distance between themselves and their offspring on several fronts. They have a stake in an ongoing situation for developmental reasons of their own.

Bengston's (1987) concept of the developmental or generational stake accounts for some of the tensions in family life. It explains why parents and children might perceive things differently. The generations are making different sets of life-changes. Parents and children have an investment or stake in their relationships that varies according to how the relationship enables the attainment of personal goals. In the case of the adolescent and her or his middle-aged parent, the parent might be concerned with the creation of a social heir while the young person is concerned with developing personal distinctiveness, a personal identity of his own (Treas & Bengston 1987).

Families consist of more than parents and children. Siblings, siblings' children, grandparents and their children's children, all are involved in the family system. Siblings play a vital role in the experience of "family", particularly for childless people. Nephews and nieces become substitute offspring, and unmarried siblings provide services that may make the difference between disruption and survival for the younger nuclear family in crisis. This, indeed, was one of the expected roles of the maiden aunt in the Victorian family (Allen 1989). Warmth between siblings is expressed both directly and indirectly. Sending Christmas and birthday presents to nephews and nieces demonstrates interest, concern and generally (though not always) affection. Present-giving involves a recognition of the younger generation but is interpreted as a gesture towards their parents as well. The notion of reciprocity binds the adults concerned, rather than the children. Remembering and forgetting birthdays is not a trivial affair but one arousing strong feelings, as symbolic aspects of family maintenance. Gestures to each other's children play a part in sustaining the links within a generation possibly weakened by the centrifugal forces of adulthood or the death of an elderly kinkeeper.

A special relationship often exists between an adult and his or her siblings' children. It is a relationship of privilege (both treats, presents and the kind of playful rudeness that anthropologists call privileged disrespect), of solidarity (aunts and uncles are sometimes the best advocates in relation to parents) and material support (aunts and uncles often act as substitute parents in times of crisis). A Mass Observation writer tells how her aunts and uncles were not in regular contact but when her cousin ran away, her father's six brothers and five sisters congregated at her house and all the men went out to look for her.

The emotional bonding of siblings and siblings' children in some ways resembles that of grandparents. Neither set of adults faces the responsibilities of parenthood and their relationships are liberated from some of its constraints.

Grandparenthood

Grandparents have been labelled "family watchdogs" (Troll 1986). They act as monitors on the sidelines of family life, prepared to act if needed, as in supporting grandchildren when their parents divorce.

In a range of situations grandparents have a beneficial influence. Studies repeatedly find that grandmothers, particularly maternal, are the most important. The grandmother–granddaughter role is particularly strong. Paternal grandfather–grandson dyads unfortunately occur much less frequently than other combinations, because men die younger than women, men become grandparents older than women, and paternal grandparents are more likely to become distanced from grandchildren following a son's divorce. (On the impact of divorce in general, see Troll 1986, Uhlenberg & Myers 1986.)

The character of grandparenthood has changed in some respects over the years. The reasons are partly demographic. In five-generational families there may be two sets of grandparent–grandchild relationships: the person in the middle can be both grandparent and grandchild simultaneously. Hagestad quotes an incident at a family gathering in which a child called out "grandma" and women from three generations responded (Hagestad 1985). Younger grandparents (in some families the role typically starts in the late thirties) are often actively involved in their younger relatives' lives. To some extent the role interferes with the pursuit of new mid-life opportunities, and young retired grandparents report feeling exploited by adult children who take their availability for granted. Presumably, work roles have the same capacity to interfere with attachment relationships at this stage as in earlier adulthood; grandparents with heavy work commitments might be less capable of building up the bank of love (Stevenson 1980) that sustains relationships between the generations when frailty disturbs the balance of give and take. However, there seems to be relatively little evidence of the narcissistic tendencies that Kornhaber claimed were invading family life and destroying grandparents' attachment to younger generations (Kornhaber 1985). Indeed, grandparents of all ages engage in mutual exchanges, their content depending on health, geographical proximity, material and other resources.

In terms of family continuity, grandparents play a vital role. They stabilize the family when it rocks, particularly by supporting the mother of the family in crisis. They have been found to be important in the transition of parenthood, both directly in providing support and indirectly in having furnished the new parent with a model of child-rearing. There is a link between new parents' own childhood and their capacity to parent (Ruoppila 1991). This extends to the pattern of attachment itself, with the parent repeating her own attachment biography (Vermulst et al. 1991).

The inheritance of a family culture and mode of living is an important influence on the young parent's capacity to cope. The experience of young families caught in the contemporary housing trap can, like attachment behaviour, be understood in a multi-generational framework. In the British public housing sector, young parents struggle to bring up families in cramped council flats, just as their grandparents struggled in tiny city-centre back-to-backs. The generation in between benefited from the large scale council house building programme of the 1950s and 1960s. Men and women raising children in flats were themselves raised, almost without exception, in houses. The young families are venturing into uncharted territory. "They carry with them the maps given to them by a previous generation, but these maps are dangerously out of date and in a lot of cases can bring only a sense of failure" (Extract from *Parenting under pressure*, reported in *Guardian*, 19 February 1992). In these circumstances, grandparents might help to counteract the feeling of failure by passing on their own skills for living.

Grandparents deflate the intensity of nuclear family interactions, partly by listening sympathetically to each protagonist in turn. Adolescents, in particular, may find in grandmothers a source of moral support. The following extract from a newspaper article (*Independent*, 20 April 1992) reflects the popular view of alternative generations as having a special bond:

> I really feel at ease with her. I take my girlfriend round there and she is quite happy about us sleeping together . . . whereas my dad still makes us sleep in separate rooms. She is very relaxed about sex and stuff. . . . It is great to be able to go round and complain about home or about dad being ridiculous or whatever. She will always be lovely and agree how stupid he is.

The grandparent–grandchild relationship is advancing in academic research, as demographic shifts turn it into a prominent feature of family life. Grandparenthood, like parenthood itself, is an increasingly common experience (Hagestad 1985, Gibson 1990, Jerrome 1993a). Given increased life expectancy, a particular relationship can last for many decades: perhaps 50 years. The emphasis since the 1960s has been on the positive aspects of the relationship – the themes arising out of the subjective experience of grandparenting, the benefits and sense of family continuity derived by grandchildren.

Interestingly, the role played by grandparents in fomenting family disputes, in dividing and ruling the next generation and in perpetuating destructive family cultures, has so far been tackled only by novelists.

Grandparents themselves experience acute frustration at times. Their contact with their grandchildren – in the dominant culture at least – is contingent on the children who give birth to them and regulate access to them. The grief of separation brought about by family breakups is often private and unremarked. It has achieved a higher profile in attempts to safeguard grandparents' rights through changes in the law. The Children Act 1989 redresses the balance by giving grandparents and other relatives the right to apply to the court to care for the child whose parents divorce. Pressure groups of grandparents in Britain concerned with access to children in a variety of situations have made themselves heard (see for instance the report, *What's in it for grandparents?*, produced by the Grandparents' Federation). The power of grandparents within the family depends partly on the family culture – the extent to which their spontaneous involvement is defined as help or interference, how much agreement there should be and sharing of problems. There are possibly ethnic variations here. Cherlin & Furstenberg (1985) found that the black grandparents in their sample were more authoritative and influential than the whites.

Similarity and consensus

Family closeness is not related to family similarities (Troll & Stapley 1985). Families can be close while disagreeing profoundly on a range of issues. But similarity of values, attitudes and outlook on the world is an important dimension of intergenerational solidarity.

Concerns about the degree of consensus between parents and children peaked as a result of the cultural movements of the 1960s, and the discussion of a generation gap. Research in the 1970s and 1980s tended to focus on attitudes, typically views of society at large. Comparisons were made of differences in the importance attached to religion, the environment, foreign policy, employment, liberalism, radicalism – a world outside the family. It was recognized that different cohorts occupy different slots in history, acquiring a particular identity and sense of shared destiny. Mention was made of a "generational keynote theme" – that distinctive set of preoccupations and orientations to the world by which generations become marked. The cognitive gap is still an issue in academic work (Bengston 1989) and in popular culture: in *The Oldie* magazine it is celebrated.

In family research, the attitudes of three generations have been compared across a range of issues. The aims of the early studies were to see how different were the attitudes of elderly parents and their adult children, middle-aged parents and their young adult children, and the first and third generations, and whether the degree of similarity changed with age or over time. Some differences were manifest across three domains – political ideology, gender ideology and religious ideology – with gender showing the greatest contrasts (Glass et al. 1986). In older dyads the adult children tend to influence their elders. In one domain in particular, that of gender ideology, the transmission of ideas appears to travel in an upward direction only.

Such attitude studies are not very revealing about the continuity of family experience. It is perhaps misguided to seek evidence of the transmission of ideas from old to young, or the extent to which people in different generations replicate each other. Given that family members have different histories and life issues to contend with it makes better sense, as Hagestad (1987) points out, to see how they manage to compromise. Family continuity requires that its members find common groups, not that they try to convert each other to sets of generation-specific beliefs.

This, indeed, is what happens. When families seek to find common ground for relating across the generations, the critical question may not be how to think about certain issues but what to think about at all. "Families vary a great deal in what they consider worthy of attention – what they think should be taken seriously. They expend a great deal of effort on finding a set of concerns that engages all of them but that is not likely to bring out differences great enough to be disruptive" (Hagestad 1987). The acceptable topics might be sports or the environment, political issues or money. Families have mechanisms for avoiding difficult issues, "demilitarized zones", silent agreements about what not to discuss.

For grandfathers and fathers in Hagestad's Chicago study, comfortable topics included work, education and finances. Women, by contrast, concentrated attention on relationships within the family, as specialists in internal family dynamics. Sore spots also varied by gender. Race relations, social policy and sex roles were touchy subjects when talking with fathers and grandfathers. With mothers and grandmothers, troublespots were topics related to interpersonal issues. These findings are similar to European studies.

The sharpest contrasts in attitudes across the generations, and potentially the most intractable, are found in immigrant families. Studies of older Jewish immigrants in California (Myerhoff 1978), London (Hazan 1980) and both USA and Britain (Francis 1984) indicate the problematic nature of relationships between the generations. In other groups, too, the elders are the alienated victims of their children's upward mobility. Cultural assimilation is compounded by social class. The older female Japanese American often finds herself without the company of her family. Her response to her social isolation varies according to whether she believes the condition is under control or might get worse; whether she interprets her daughter's absence as part of her motherly duty to care for her child rather than neglectful of her parent; whether her daughter agrees with her on other important matters; and whether she actually has a desire for close interpersonal ties in the first place (Osako & Liu 1986). In fact, in practice the norm of filial piety remains strong, in Asian cultures in Britain as well as the USA. For the less fortunate elders who are alienated from their successful offspring, a variety of strategies on group goals and dependence on the ethnic group as a whole helps older people to accept their reduced status in relation to their offspring.

Nonetheless, this experience draws our attention back to the issue of the generational stake. This was the suggestion that the developmental needs of older and younger family members – one for generativity, the other for identity – are incompatible. The idea of the generational stake helps to account not just for the distress of older immigrant parents but for the reluctance of parents to acknowledge that their children are on the brink of divorce. It underlies the bitterness of older women whose daughters fail to follow their example of full-time home making and church work, choosing instead to work for money and pay someone else to look after their children (Jerrome 1992).

Ideas about the family

As these examples suggest, a major area of discontinuity in ideas is the family itself. Norms and expectations concerning family life vary across the generations. Differences range from definitions of who to regard as "family" to how relatives should be treated. Sociologists describe the contemporary western family as less regulated by social norms than in earlier decades. They suggest that there is more room for manoeuvre and individual negotiation of rules. Social historians such as Edward Shorter (1977), for instance, argue that an emphasis on duty as a basis for family involvement has given way to one on preference and liking. The main unit for identification – the nuclear family – is typically small and structurally unsupported.

The evidence of the Mass Observation Archive suggests that the contemporary image of the small, isolated nuclear family is misleading in several respects. In relation to the numbers of people involved in "the family", for instance, there are substantial variations in the perceived scope of this unit. Today's young nuclear family is likely to be linked to several others by active bonds of kinship. Despite the change in size of household unit, strong emotional bonds still exist between adult siblings and the ascending and descending generations. There is, however, a strong sense that people are more selective these days about who they keep in touch with. One writer, fascinated by the contrast between the Victorian family photo expressing solidarity and uniformity with the present fragmented family of her experience, writes:

> these days contact depends on liking, judgements on whether they are nice or not, their relative earning power, interests. My own criterion is, would I visit a relative if I were passing their door? No. Would I send a present to a cousin in Marriage? No, I don't like her and she earns more than me. Who would I visit? A cousin with a similar lifestyle: if she lived next door we'd be friends.

It is indeed a case of personal preference and mutual attraction, but not entirely. A popular saying to the effect that you choose your friends but are saddled with your relatives (variously attributed to George Bernard Shaw, Hilaire Beloc and Walt Whitman) is frequently invoked. It implies that relatives exist whether you like them or not: that people go on being involved even though they do not get on. The saying is invoked to account for coolness and a reluctance to ask for help from kin. It is used most frequently by people who prefer their friends to their relatives and feel the need to justify it.

The Mass Observation material presents very different ideas of who and what the family is. There seem to be two main ways of conceptualizing it. One is to include everyone known to be linked by blood and marriage, with various limits set by time and degrees of kinship. The other is to define it in terms of contact, as a unit based on affect. Such a definition is seen as lacking in logic, and certainly it involves a different kind of logic from the reckoning of formal kinship.

People who think of family as genealogy often start by saying what a difficult task it is to define "relatives". Should one include just one's own relatives or those of one's husband as well? What about those of both sets of parents? People typically don't know how many they have and set about counting them up. One such woman came up with 51 own relatives, 83 in-laws, and 9 offspring, making 143 altogether. She has no contact with most of them. Others count their relatives in hundreds. For instance, "200 relatives on my mother's side, 79 of them in regular contact, and 55 exchanging regular visits with me".

Even widely dispersed units of the family are counted if they are known. The impact of emigration in earlier decades of the century and before makes the task more difficult, but links with relatives in North America, Southern Africa, Australasia and the Middle East are common.

For a woman born in 1924, with 90 relatives including in-laws and third cousins spread over four generations, "the family" has clarity and firmness. It is conceived in the form of a pyramid with traceable lines of descent and lateral ties created by marriage; membership is recorded in volumes of named photographs. She is not alone among Mass Observation respondents in attaching importance to the family name itself, threatened when a particular generation contains more girls than boys. Family gatherings are important ritual occasions.

The concept of *family as a unit based on affect* is quite different. For a social worker born in 1928, "Relatives are people related by blood whom I know and like. They are NOT people I neither know nor like." The number of relatives in this case is small. A select number of them – favourite cousins and sisters-in-law – are given special ritual status, invited to be godparents to her daughters.

The notion of family as affect ignores formal kinship. It ranges far and wide, however, going beyond the nuclear family. A young woman born in 1950 lists as her family relatives who are remote in kinship terms – "sort of step-second cousins, I think" (mother's mother's half-brother's daughter's daughters). In addition to these young women who belong to her generation but have a common ancestor four generations back, she includes her husband's father's father's second wife and her son by a previous marriage, and the son's children.

These two folk models of kinship correspond to the contrasting models used by anthropologists – the ancestor-focused unit of social structure, and ego-focused kindred. Both ways of conceptualizing the family, it would seem, reflect the reality of contemporary experience (Strathern 1992, Jerrome 1994a). Ideas about the scope of the family vary between families and within the same family. That they change over the generations is evident from accounts offered by middle-aged people of the different perceptions of their children, and by those of adults whose parents disagree with their definitions. However, the direction of change is not predictable. The conventional sociological model of family change from one type to another seems, in the light of Mass Observation evidence, to overemphasize the shifts in social structure and ignore the elements of continuity over time.

Implicit in the acceptance of people as kin is an understanding of a certain quality of relationship. Being "family" involves a certain kind of behaviour, and on this dimension too, the generations – generally parents and children but sometimes uncles and aunts and nephews and nieces – disagree. These intergenerational differences are often a source of tension and disappointment. The lack of consensus is evident in the following extract:

> We can see a difference in our grandparents' and parents' atti-
> tudes towards "family". We have a more relaxed, informal
> approach and accept that all relatives are individuals, some of
> whom are more appealing than others! We keep in close contact
> with those we love and have something in common with and
> have little to do with the others. Over the years, I have watched
> older relatives see them as they have endured the company of
> relatives they positively dislike merely because they are "fam-
> ily" and duty visits have been expected of them.

We do not know whether in this case the difference of outlook causes trouble between the generations. In other extracts the experience of tension is clear. Family members have different expectations of family life depending on their personal needs. These expectations are based partly on recollections of a more satisfactory situation some time in the person's past. They are justified also by reference to what are perceived as universal ideas of what "the family" is all about.

Disappointment is accounted for in personal theories of change and decline in the family as an institution (Jerrome 1994a). These folk theories emphasize affluence, materialism, and a general decline in family responsibilities.

When family members need different things there is tension. When needs coincide, family members are fortunate. The differences are not entirely predictable, nor are they inevitably age linked. An elderly man writes with gratitude of the younger generation whose commitment to "the family" is stronger than his was. He talks of the growing social distance between himself and his siblings, a "drifting apart" for which there was no reason, which followed no rift. His younger relatives are trying to restore ties that his generation "had allowed to drop away". He recognizes the benefit to his sons of newly discovered kin, and appreciates for himself the growing attachment to his own elderly sister.

An explanation for his sons' revival of interest in kinship may be found at different levels: the current boom in the pursuit of genealogy as a cultural phenomenon, the cult of heritage, the personal need of young parents for a sense of family continuity and historical depth, the psychological transition from the pursuit of intimacy to the need for generativity (Jerome 1996).

Conclusion: the future

Families are groups of people in more or less intimate relationship, interacting, forming attachments, and sharing ideas. The variability of experience in the realm of family life that emerges from personal accounts contradicts the suggestion of more general age-linked and historical trends in the literature. "Family" appears to be a continuing and vital dimension of experience. In terms of changes in the family as an institution, some historical trends seem clear. It has become increasingly necessary, for instance, to separate the concept of "family" from that of "household" in a society that is ageing, and prone to divorce and remarriage (Hagestad 1987). We have tended to assume that household composition provided a clue to family composition. In the twenty-first century we might expect even greater diversity as rates of divorce and remarriage accelerate and formal kinship becomes even less closely associated with intimate living arrangements.

New key dyads in addition to the current ones of parent–child and husband–wife might appear. Vertical links between grandparents, grandchildren and even great-grandchildren are likely to become a stronger feature of family relationships, assuming that current demographic trends continue. Equally, horizontal ties between siblings are likely to increase in importance as sibling groups grow old together (Jerrome 1991, 1993a). As horizontal bonds between siblings are sustained, so the vertical ties between siblings and siblings' children are reinforced, with implications for family continuity.

The growth in complexity indicates the need for a more flexible concept of the family. This is in keeping with the currently critical approach towards certain other social constructs. Traditional age categories, for instance, have been modified to take account of changing age norms and possibilities. It is appropriate that the family, which is a major context for ageing, should be subject to the same critical scrutiny.

CHAPTER 5

Obligations and support within families

Hazel Qureshi

Be wise you parents, yield not yourselves captives and prison-
ers to your children; no prison can be more irksome to a parent
than a son or daughter's house. (Daniel Rogers 1642, quoted in
Thomas 1976)

Introduction

How will the ageing of the population affect the provision of care and
support within families? As will be indicated, policy-makers and
practitioners operate on a variety of assumptions about family obligations and these may or may not be accurate. This chapter will draw on
a wealth of evidence and commentary about who gives what to
whom, and on what terms, in order to describe accurately present patterns of support and generate an understanding of the underlying factors that bring these about. Of course, other features of the social and
economic context will be changing along with the age structure of the
population, and whilst it not possible to predict these changes in
detail, they have to be considered in discussing possible changes in
family obligations. This chapter begins with a brief discussion of the
family and the state and goes on to outline some of the available evidence, first about patterns of support and second about underlying
factors. Likely implications for the future are then considered in the
light of expected demographic changes that mean greater numbers of
older people and relatively fewer potential family carers.

Family help and state help

Clearly the state has an interest in the provision of care by families, and the policies of the state will have direct and indirect effects on the provision of such care. Coercion is one method that may be used to make sure care is provided (for example prosecution for neglect of children), but, as outlined in the Introduction to this volume, this method has largely proved unsuccessful in relation to the care of older relatives. Incentives such as tax allowances and benefits are also possible methods to induce people to care for dependent relatives. Land (1978) has noted how the construction of social policy in Britain has been affected by the desire to strike an appropriate balance between the perceived danger of allowing the state to take on too many responsibilities, thus weakening family ties, as opposed to offering too little help thus causing the family to collapse under the unrelieved burden of providing care. Of course the need to restrict public expenditure may also be a reason for not wishing to take over responsibilities from the family but the "rightness" of the primacy of family help is often emphasized (see for example Griffiths 1988).

The belief that state help drives out family help and that the provision of help is related to the strength of family ties has not been of such concern in all European countries. Waerness (1990) argues from Norwegian experience that assistance is not a "zero-sum" game, but rather that the growth in public care systems was necessary because the need for care outstripped the capacity of the family to provide it. In addition the public services enabled older people to achieve the intimacy at a distance, which they preferred to characterize family relationships, even after they became disabled. Siim (1990) comments that elderly people in Denmark prefer to receive state help which they see as a right of citizenship. The way in which services are organized and provided, and the assumptions made about the responsibilities of families will influence the provision of family care. In addition the general economic and social conditions within a particular country will influence capacity of families to provide care for each other.

Policy and evidence about family and informal support
In 1981 a Government White Paper on care for older people observed "the primary sources of support and care for older people are informal and voluntary" thus acknowledging the lesser contribution of statutory services. Unfortunately, the White Paper then went on to

101

misidentify the basis on which most informal care is provided: "These spring from the personal ties of friendship and neighbourhood" (DHSS 1981: 3) thus failing to recognize that informal care was overwhelmingly care by kin. Perhaps this is part of the explanation why the knowledge that most care was informal seemed to become translated at first into a perception that there was an untapped pool of informal helpers in the community that might be drawn on to replace expensive statutory care.

> The personal social services provide only a small part of the totality of care in the community for . . . the elderly, the old and frail, the physically handicapped and the mentally ill. . . . When one is comparing where one can make savings . . . in personal social services there is a substantial possibility and, indeed, probability of continuing growth in the amount of voluntary care, of neighbourhood care, of self-help. (Secretary of State for Social Services 1980)

Throughout the 1980s a number of studies of elderly people were conducted that focused not only on people giving care but also on the whole informal network. These indicated that the community, particularly the family, was working at full capacity, and that there was no slack in the system that could easily be utilized (Wenger 1984, 1992, Qureshi & Walker 1989). How this may be concluded from this work will be indicated later. These studies, whilst not national, covered both urban and rural areas, and focused on representative community-based samples of elderly people. At the same time, national data on carers that became available during the 1980s made it clear just how much greater was the contribution of kin compared with other possible sources of informal help (Green 1988, Arber & Ginn 1990, 1991), and reinforced the message of earlier British and North American work that the amount of informal care provided in the community far outweighed the amount of statutory care.

In addition to this improved knowledge base, a range of feminist authors produced a stream of work that was critical of unequal gender divisions in caring, and of the extent to which policy and services played a part in reproducing disadvantage for women (for example Finch & Groves 1980, 1983, Ungerson 1987). This literature emphasized the stresses and strains imposed on women who gave care, and the essentially compulsory nature of their apparent altruism in a context where there were no suitable alternative services (Land & Rose 1985, Finch 1987). In addition at this time, carers' organizations campaigned to draw attention to the need for adequate support services to help those who were giving care. Although the arguments of these two groups often reinforced each other their central concerns were different, as feminists wanted a de-emphasizing of the family as the central feature of community care (Finch 1990), whilst carers tended to stress their willingness to care given the right support (Evidence to House of Commons Social Services Committee, session 1989–90). Both groups probably contributed along with a number of studies of carers (Equal Opportunities Commission 1980, Nissel & Bonnerjea 1982) to reinforcing the idea of the typical carer as being a middle-aged woman. What was principally lacking in this period was any detailed understanding of the preferences and wishes of elderly people themselves with regard to sources of care. The assumption that elderly people would prefer family care seemed to hold sway and was supported by the work of Abrams (1978) who argued that care from informal sources such as family members was experienced as superior because it was evidence that people personally cared about the person receiving it.

Again some of the evidence and argument seemed to have influence although there was little comfort from policy-makers for the feminist point of view. In 1989, introducing the government's White Paper on Community Care, the Secretary of State said:

the great bulk of community care will continue, as now, to be provided by family, friends and neighbours. The majority of carers take on these responsibilities willingly, and I admire the dedicated and self-sacrificing way in which so many members of the public take on serious obligations to help care for elderly or disabled relatives and friends. Our proposals are aimed at strengthening support for those many unselfish people who care for people in need. (House of Commons Hansard 1493 col 976)

Thus the emphasis has shifted from increasing care by the community towards maintaining and preserving it. As Twigg (1989) observed it had become clear that informal care, whilst of key importance, was not a "commandable resource". The White Paper described practical support for carers as a key objective for service delivery, but also revealed an expectation that this would prove a value-for-money approach, arguing that "helping carers maintain their valuable contribution to the spectrum of care is both right and a sound investment" (para 2.3).

What patterns of support exist within families?

The flows of support and help among families take many different forms. People can exchange emotional support, material goods or cash, or practical help. Assistance within this system is personally directed, that is, it is given by virtue of pre-existing social or biological relationships. In this respect, as Abrams (1978) indicated, it differs from care as distributed through the formal statutory or voluntary systems, which aim to distribute resources to people in predefined categories of need, and to give most to those in most need. If we consider what is known, for example, about the distribution of financial and material assistance across the generations it is clear that this is undertaken to improve the relative life chances of those who are personally linked. A study limited to Sheffield (Qureshi & Simons 1987) gave results consistent with earlier work (Bell 1968) and demonstrated that the exchange of material resources was influenced by the relative needs and affluence of the two generations. The overall effect of intergenerational flows was towards equalizing resources between generations but this occurred largely within social classes. Relatives identified as unemployed, recently redundant, sick or disabled were least likely to be receiving any financial assistance from parents. It is worthwhile to consider the example of financial help before moving on to look at practical assistance and personal care, because it illustrates some features of the informal system that are of relevance to considering how it meshes in with the formal statutory or voluntary system. First, the overall distribution that is the outcome of the family system is not towards those with the greatest needs; secondly, those with equal needs do not receive equal help.

The context in which need for care arises

At any one time most elderly people do not require care, although this does not necessarily mean that they will not be receiving informal domestic assistance: 37 per cent of non-disabled men identified in the 1985 General Household Survey were receiving such assistance (Arber & Ginn 1991). Other data from this survey indicated that among people aged over 64, 14 per cent of women were severely disabled compared with 7 per cent of men. As well as the greater likeli-hood that they will suffer disabling diseases, women generally face a different context to men in terms of the capacity for generating inten-sive informal assistance: 75 per cent of older men are married com-pared with 40 per cent of older women. In higher age groups these disparities increase. Two-thirds of severely disabled elderly men receive personal and domestic care from their wives, whereas a minor-ity of equally disabled women receive help from husbands (28 per cent receive personal care, 20 per cent domestic care). This is a consequence of several factors but primarily gender differences in life expectancy. It is this kind of evidence that has led some authors to suggest that women's greater involvement in "kinkeeping" activities of the kind described by Rosenthal (1985), makes sense from the point of view of self-interest (Spitze & Logan 1989).

Evidence about who provides care

As Arber & Ginn (1990) observe there are a number of caveats about the data from the OPCS survey of informal carers (Green 1988). Never-theless this is the best nationally representative data available about carers and it provides a useful overall framework of information that has plausibly suggested that a number of prevailing assumptions about the distribution of care need a correction of emphasis. Table 5.1 shows the sources of informal care for older people (aged 65+). It demonstrates the difference in distribution of sources that is obtained by looking at the numbers of carers as opposed to the amount of care provided by them. Friends and neighbours are 22 per cent of carers but they provide only 7 per cent of the total care.

The majority (61 per cent) of hours of care come from people in the same household as the elderly person, although 80 per cent of carers live in another household. On average co-resident carers provide 53

Table 5.1 Sources of informal care.

Care-provider	Per cent of care-givers	Per cent of hours of care
Spouse	8	30
Child	39	40
Child-in-law	14	11
Other relative	18	12
Friend or neighbour	22	7

Source: Arber & Ginn, 1991: Table 8.2

hours per week, compared with 9 hours per week for out-of-household carers. Arber and Ginn (1990, 1991) argue from this that the contribution made by older people themselves to providing care has been neglected, and that the perception of older people as passive recipients of care needs to be revised. Many studies have indicated that statutory services go overwhelmingly to people who live alone, and Wenger (1990) on the basis of studies of elderly people in Wales, had already observed the failure of services to develop sensitive interventions for working with elderly caring spouses. It was clear that the neglect of spouses also meant a neglect of a substantial group of male carers (Arber & Gilber 1989). How much of the total care for older people was provided by the stereotypical middle-aged female carer?

Table 5.2   Providers of care (per cent of total hours per week).

Age	Gender of carer		Total
	Male	Female	
Under 45	8	16	24
45–64	13	28	41
65+	16	19	35
Total	37	63	100

Source: Arber & Ginn, 1991: Table 8.3

Middle-aged women were providing 28 per cent of the total care to older people. Of course this is an underestimate of the demands made on them in their capacity as carers, since these women in the middle generation may also be providing care to disabled children. Analysis of the data not restricted to elderly people showed that care for a disabled child was 17 per cent of all informal care (Arber & Ginn 1990) and available evidence suggests this is largely provided by women (Parker 1990). In addition, as Wenger (1990) suggests, the existing balance of relationships suffers a greater disturbance for younger women caring, whilst for elderly spouses caring is more likely to be the focus of their lives. Pollitt et al. (1991) also report this in relation to spouses caring for elderly people with dementia, although they, like Wenger, argue that certain forms of service intervention could be valuable in assisting people in this situation. So then perhaps the greater focus on women in the middle reflects their greater opportunity costs in caring, as well as the particular meaning of caring to spouses.

In looking at the stresses of caring within joint households one key distinction emerges in many studies. This is whether the formation of the household predated dependency, or occurred as a consequence of dependency. The second situation is universally found to be more stressful (Arber & Gilbert 1989), with carers in long established joint households better able to cope and more anxious to keep their relatives at home (Wenger 1992). From this Wenger argues that incentives to encourage the formation of shared households for frail elderly parents are unlikely to work in the long term and therefore probably would not be cost-effective (p. 204), although intensive assistance to keep elderly people in life-long joint households would be much appreciated.

In longitudinal work Wenger (1992) has demonstrated that people who need personal care are unlikely to remain in the community unless they have within-household care from a close relative. A descriptive typology of support networks has been developed that reflects the degree to which the person has access to support from local kin, distant kin, neighbours and friends (Wenger 1989) and it is argued that the distribution of network types is related to characteristics of the community, particularly levels of in and out-migration and, to a lesser extent, population density (Wenger & St Leger 1992). In relation to the degree to which additional informal support might be generated for older people Wenger argues that her studies, conducted in both urban and rural areas show that:

> some networks . . . can be counted on to provide a high level of committed informal support in old age, while others have no likelihood of informal care in the face of growing dependency and loss of reciprocity. (Wenger 1992: 191)

At low levels of dependency where needs are for routine support at low levels of frequency, and for emotional support, many people can find this within their local community. However, only certain networks can respond to high levels of dependency requiring personal care and other help at short intervals. Given this, Wenger argues that expectations of generating more informal help for highly dependent people who do not receive it spontaneously are unrealistic. Effectively, the type and level of care available to people depends on the normative expectations associated with the particular members of their informal network, and the informal care system cannot be made to work outside these. The next section will consider in detail what these obligations are and from whence they arise.

The basis of family obligations in Britain

We have seen that routine informal practical support and personal care for elderly people are primarily a matter for close kin in practice, although relatives other than spouses or children, as well as friends and neighbours, are involved in a limited way. On what basis is this care provided? Do people subscribe to common ideas about the responsibility of kin, or are patterns of behaviour and belief varying and changing? Finch and Mason (1990) investigated the degree to which there was a consensus among a random sample of the population in the north-west of England about obligations between adult kin (see also Ch. 6). This survey did find that the majority of people gave general assent to the idea of filial obligations applying in a range of possible situations where need for care might be envisaged. However, this support for obligations of children must be qualified by the observation that in a majority of cases people had opted for a solution other than family care as a first choice (Finch & Mason 1990: 156). In other societies, where different material conditions prevail, the expectation of direct reciprocation from children once parents reach old age may be much clearer, reflecting at least partly a perceived lack of alternative sources of care. Part of the campaign to encourage adherence to the One-Child Programme in China has been the promotion of older people's residential facilities (Harper 1992). However, it is doubtful that children in western industrial society are a good financial investment for their parents' old age, nor are the returns guaranteed. The older generation, as Finch (1989) observed from a review of the literature, are the net givers over the life-cycle, and the preferred state is of independence and a continuing capacity to assist one's children into old age. Overall the desirable scenario is that parents are able to remain net givers over the life-time and to preserve their independence and "intimacy at a distance" that separate households but affectionate relationships can supply.

Qureshi and Walker (1989) in a study of caring relatives found that those who experienced particular difficulties in their own caring relationships were most inclined to wish to offer qualifications and add conditions to general statements about obligations. In this latter study the idea of a hierarchy of obligations was used to explore actual patterns of provision of regular practical domestic, and in some cases personal, care. Relatives appeared to be largely chosen in accordance with a hierarchy that was: spouse, relative living in the household, daughter, daughter-in-law, son, other relative or neighbour. Interviews with carers confirmed that there were corresponding normative beliefs in operation, so that where for example, relatives were not chosen in accordance with this hierarchy then an explanation was offered to legitimize this, or conflict within the network was reported. Choices in accordance with this hierarchy did not have to be explained, indeed when asked for an explanation as to why they helped, relatives were sometimes taken aback, and could not understand the meaning of the question or offered a simple statement of the relationship: "I am her daughter". It was felt that this particular hierarchy of choices was produced from an interaction between beliefs about the responsibilities of close kin, and beliefs about the gender-appropriateness of the particular tasks under consideration. Thus hierarchy for personal care might be structured differently, perhaps with a same-sex child preferred, so that sons might be expected to assist widowed fathers. Similarly a hierarchy for providing financial help might concentrate on male relatives. It can be seen how such hierarchies could vary across cultures, and within cultures over time, as ideas about gender roles changed.

The importance of ideas about gender roles in shaping the hierarchy demonstrates a potential for intergenerational conflict if these ideas are changing. For example, cross-generational differences in gender expectations related to housework were reported to have caused conflict in a number of Sheffield families. Elderly widowed men sometimes expected a level of domestic servicing that their daughters and daughters-in-law were not accustomed to provide within their own household, and there were situations where elderly women and men discouraged help that crossed traditional gender boundaries. Services have been criticized for showing gender bias because domiciliary care seemed to be given to men at lower levels of disability than women (Qureshi & Walker 1989, Waerness 1990) and because female carers were given different combinations of services to male carers (Charlesworth et al. 1984). Detailed analysis of national data suggested that gender differences in service receipt were not as great as had been supposed by earlier commentators, once account had been taken of the different circumstances in which elderly women and men were living, although the distribution of domiciliary care and meals on wheels seemed to show some gender bias (Arber et al. 1988).

Since it has been shown that relatives play a part in securing statutory care, and indeed that people with no relatives may sometimes be disadvantaged when it comes to the receipt of services (Davies & Challis 1986, Waerness 1990), it is of interest that people in Sheffield who had sons only were more likely to be receiving home help than people with no children. This highlights an important point: where services are in short supply, people without family to advocate on their behalf may be less likely to obtain them. The obligations of children to "see that parents are all right" do not have to include personal performance of the tasks, although there are separate obligations to maintain contact that do have to be personally discharged. Therefore, if changing social conditions increase conflict about who should help, then families may seek to resolve this by seeking public services.

Working out who should help in practice

Finch & Mason (1990) in their exploration of a case study of a family deciding who should help an elderly relative, agree that a hierarchy of obligations is appealed to by the actors involved, but suggest that whether the expectations generated will be translated into particular actions depends on a range of normative guidelines that include: the quality of the personal relationship; considerations of reciprocity; the appropriate "time of life"; and the desired balance of dependence and independence in the relationships involved. Finch (1989 and Ch. 6) argues that decisions about care are further complicated by their dependence on individual understandings and commitments that are specific to the history of the particular relationship. The negotiation of care in these terms becomes a complex and tricky business. There is much support for this framework from the comments of the carers in Sheffield although many of these factors will not come into play in most instances in the way that they do in the case study Finch and Mason describe (where there were six children), because there are few people to choose from: only one in three people over 74 in Sheffield had a family that contained at least one son and one daughter. The general scope for complex negotiations should not be overestimated. But the following discussion of some of the findings illustrates how normative beliefs about gender roles are also brought in to play and illustrate some of the scope for intergenerational conflict in working out the proper thing to do.

110

Our work would suggest that the quality of the relationship is unlikely to be easily accepted as a reason for failure to help elderly parents. Certainly people helped despite reporting past and present poor relationships (Qureshi 1986), and some children who were not keen to help described ways in which other people such as neighbours, the police and social services had actively conveyed to them an expectation that they were expected to do so (Qureshi & Walker 1989). The expectation that obligation to parents would be reinforced by a personal sense of debt to them was not met in these instances. "She's never been a mother as mothers should be" explained a son-in-law. The situation in which people felt obliged to help parents towards whom they felt no sense of personal obligation was experienced as stressful "if I could think of a few good things my mother had done for me it would make it easy, it would make it a lot easier" said one daughter. Nevertheless these helpers had found the obligation to help compelling. However, there were indications that the willingness to help in such circumstances did not extend to a preparedness to form a joint household in the event of severe disability.

In studies of people caring for relatives with dementia the reported quality of the past relationship and a lack of emotional closeness have been linked to the expressed willingness on the part of the carer to accept residential care by Gilhooley (1986) and Levin et al. (1986) respectively, and these expressed attitudes are predictive of eventual admission. The obligations of marriage may be even stronger in this respect. Pollitt et al. (1991: 465) found that the "balance of compensations and satisfactions" among spouses caring for dementia sufferers depended on the previous relationship, although those who seemed to help only out of resignation or duty expressed willingness to carry on caring, despite a lower likelihood of experiencing caring as rewarding. In the case study described by Finch and Mason a woman estranged from her elderly husband was subject to, and succumbed to, expectations that she should provide care for him when he became disabled.

In contrast, the quality of the relationship and the history of reciprocity with people outside the close kin group can mean that individuals can be "defined in" and will be treated as if they were kin. The long-term history of the relationship is of key importance in such instances. Anything more than routine help to neighbours depends on the existence of long-established relationships in which clear patterns of reciprocity have been enjoyed that involve the previous

111

giving of help beyond the normal bounds of neighbourliness. More distant kin who had played a parenting role could also be defined in. This basis for the generation of high levels of help to more distant relatives or neighbours is not something that can be created at or after the point of dependency. Thus even though neighbours and friends provide a small proportion of care there is little likelihood of generating an increase to care for more dependent people.

Our understanding of how norms operate in practice can be enhanced if we consider the reasons that people regarded as legitimate excuses for not providing care. Three types of excuses were recognized as legitimate: prior obligations to other family members, the personal incapacity of the "expected" helper and the unreasonable behaviour of the person requiring care. Just as there is a hierarchy of people who may recognize an obligation to assist a particular person, so there is an order of priority among the possible demands that a person can be expected to meet. In the western industrial nations this has been observed to be: family of procreation (spouse and children); family of orientation (parents and siblings); affinal family (the family of the spouse). Clearly this order of priorities differs across cultures, for example the second two are reversed for women in cultures where they are considered to join their husband's family on marriage.

Explanations in terms of physical and mental incapacity of the expected helper are at first sight straightforward: "my sister is crippled with arthritis" said one daughter, explaining why she helped alone. There was little reported conflict around explanations reported in these terms. However, the question of gender-related ideas about capacity to help is relevant here too. One son explained that most women were able to give the kind of help that elderly people required whilst most men did not have the necessary skills to do so. "Unreasonable behaviour" normally centred round the idea that the elderly person had not been a "proper parent". The concept of reciprocity is not quite adequate to explain what is going on when people are "defined out" as being not deserving of care although previous examples will have made it clear that failure to help in the past is often involved. There could be other kinds of behaviour that children defined as not proper such as an elderly parent getting remarried "too soon" after widowhood, or expressing disapproval of the child's own divorce and remarriage.

Social and demographic changes that will influence patterns of family support

Given what is understood about current distributions of support, and the basis on which it is provided within families, it becomes possible to speculate about the likely effects of a number of structural changes that are known to be occurring. Some of these, such as the greater prevalence of multi-generational families, are clearly related to the ageing of the population. Others, such as changing patterns of divorce and remarriage, may not be, but are of importance to intergenerational obligations and support because they form a central part of the context within which these are worked out. There are of course many relevant factors about which uncertainty remains: for example the question of the likely level of need for support in relation to chronological age (Bebbington 1988, Arber & Ginn 1991: 119). Despite this uncertainty, it seems likely that women will continue to be disadvantaged compared to men in relation to disability and poor health in later life. Their lower access to material resources, and to informal caring resources that would be likely to provide intensive support, will also continue.

Multi-generational families

As Waerness (1990) observes, when parents and children are likely to experience more than 50 years of overlapping life, there will be adults on both sides of the intergenerational relationship for most of the time. It will be increasingly common for grandparent–grandchild relationships to be adult to adult. When families may contain two generations of pensioners and perhaps two generations of widows, the possible range of conflicting demands on the middle generation identified by Brody (1981, 1985) will be increasing, and the demands of providing care may affect retirement as well as working life. It may also be of importance that inheritance will be delayed, and that resources accumulated by the oldest generation may well have been largely consumed in meeting ordinary living expenses into old age, let alone by any need that might have arisen for care. Perhaps there will be larger numbers of younger relatives available as carers? At present adult grandchildren are not reported as playing a significant role in the care of their grandparents, especially once they have established independent homes, and, in working out who should give care, the care of their own young children would be an acceptable prior obligation. Grandchildren still living in their parents home and dependent upon

113

them might be seen to have an obligation to help but as a duty to their parents rather than grandparents. Women's higher levels of employment once their own children are no longer dependent mean that they are less likely to take a key role in childcare while their grandchildren are young (Anderson 1985). In individual cases particular histories may mean a grandparent becoming "defined in" as a surrogate parent but there does not seem to be a basis for a widespread expansion of care given by grandchildren.

Patterns of divorce and remarriage

Anderson (1979) points out that in pre-twentieth-century Europe, marriages were more likely to be broken in their early years than they are today, although by death rather than by divorce. He argues that many of the problems associated with marital breakup are not new, and clearly it is important not to overstate changes. Nevertheless the fact that ex-spouses remain alive and may or may not remarry does have some quite different consequences for kinship obligations and for the care of some groups of elderly people. For example there may be an increasing number of men surviving into old age but having little or no contact with their children. Spitze and Miner (1992) identified such an isolated group among black elders in the USA. Goldscheider (1990) also argued that more generally divorced men do not see their children as sources of support in later life. It seems reasonable to hypothesize an increase in the numbers of elderly divorced men with limited access to informal support.

Of course, as discussed, most older men obtain informal support if needed from their wives, and there is some limited evidence that marriages contracted later in life may not generate the same degree of commitment on the part of spouses to provide care (Wenger 1992), especially when disability is severe. Another possibility then is a decrease in the proportion of spouses who will willingly undertake long-term heavy caring tasks.

Divorce may strengthen family ties between parents and children if the divorced child returns to the parental home or is otherwise assisted by the older generation. Certainly there is evidence that people are more likely to be living with relatives after a marriage has ended than during it (Sullivan 1986). The difficulties of the situation might worsen relationships of course, but in general there would be an expectation that the sense of debt to the parents would be increased. The Sheffield study offered some evidence that effects of divorce on contact with parents differed for women and men: divorced daughters had more contact with parents than other daughters, whereas divorced sons had less contact than other sons unless they had returned to the parental home (Qureshi & Walker 1989). For daughters, therefore, the obligation to assist parents in old age may be thus strengthened or reinforced after divorce, but equally the financial consequences of divorce may well mean that the women concerned are less likely to have the time and resources to provide assistance, and more likely to have sole responsibility for children as a prior obligation.

In considering obligations within reconstituted families a number of factors will influence the degree to which a given step-relationship is treated "as if" it were a kin relationship. The affective quality of the relationship and the length of co-residence would seem likely candidates. Remarriage of an elderly person in later life could cause conflict with children, and might make it less likely that they would assist in caring for the spouse in the event of disability. It seems likely that whether a step-relationship will be treated as if it were a kin relation ship will depend on the degree to which the normal life-cycle patterns associated with the particular kin relationship have been followed. Where children may have had four or more "parent figures" in their lives it becomes difficult to sustain the idea that there will be a commitment or a capacity to provide intensive levels of help for them all. The scope for negotiation around the question of who owes what to whom becomes extremely complex.

Employment and unemployment

Several effects of women's greater participation in the labour market have been suggested. The conflict between employment and caring has figured large in discussions of the strains of upon carers (Parker 1990), and both daughters and daughters-in-law have been shown to be less likely to be providing assistance to elderly relatives if they were in full-time work (Qureshi & Walker 1989). It might be supposed that men who were unemployed would be in a position to provide greater assistance to relatives but the Sheffield study found that unemployed sons seemed to be less likely to provide practical help than employed sons. Morris (1985) pointed to a failure to renegotiate the division of domestic labour after redundancy and suggested a number of reasons for this that might also apply to unemployed sons' failure to undertake informal help for their parents. It was suggested that the assumption of responsibility for "female" tasks involves a threat to the man's gender identity that is already threatened by the loss of employment; further the quality of the husband's domestic labour compared with the wife's is likely to be poor; finally the need to be available for work militates against undertaking long-term commitments to provide care.

Wenger (1992) argues that out-migration in search of employment will have substantial effects upon the likely supply of informal help for elderly people in particular areas, thus leading either to greater needs for formal help in the event of disability, or the creation of demands for more housing suitable for elderly people in the areas to which the younger generation has moved. Moving house in this way of course will disrupt the elderly person's existing network and restrict their contacts with friends and neighbours outside the family. It may be the only way in which family obligations can be met, but it may not be the preference of the elderly person if alternative sources of care were available. Wenger noted that middle class migrants with local networks that did not include close kin were likely to use commercial help to cope with lower levels of disability and to make early requests for statutory help rather than to move to join (geographically) distant close kin.

Cultural diversity

As has been indicated, many of the features of the hierarchy of obligations and the normative guidelines within which they are translated into action will vary across different cultures. For example, within Asian families in Britain there is some evidence that joint households are more common, and certainly in a TV programme (*East*, BBC2, August 1992) Asian elders interviewed interpreted the British reluctance to share households as evidence of a lack of care for elderly people in this society. There is also evidence that daughters-in-law take precedence over daughters in deciding who should give practical assistance, as a consequence of a prevailing belief that sons rather than daughters are primarily responsible for ensuring that parents get care if needed (Cameron et al. 1989). The number of black and Asian elders is known to be increasing: available figures show only 4 per cent of people from minority ethnic groups are over pensionable age compared with 19 per cent of the white population (Arber & Ginn 1991) but this reflects the particular demographic structure of a population formed largely by in-migration during the 1950s and 1960s, and so large proportionate increases may be expected; for example, the number of Asian elders is expected to double during the 1990s. There have been many criticisms of statutory services for their failure to understand the needs and wishes of elderly people from minority ethnic groups, and of the stereotyped assumptions made by professionals about family obligations as exercised within these groups (Bhaduri & Wright 1990, Atkin 1991, 1992). Providing suitable services to help black and Asian elderly people and their family carers is, and will continue to be, a major challenge for services (Butt et al. 1991, Atkin & Rollings 1992, Wilson 1992).

Conclusion

Both historical experience and a knowledge of the basis on which obligations are based suggest that attempts to legally impose a duty to care that runs counter to prevailing beliefs about what should be properly expected would be likely to be met with evasion and passive resistance. Family obligations and intergenerational support will continue to operate and evolve according to the material circumstances, individual histories and normative beliefs of those within them. The pressures on women in the middle generation seem set to increase and there is little evidence that men in the middle will increasingly take on caring roles. Given that relatives can and do play a role in advocating for public services, and that securing such assistance may be a way of settling or avoiding conflict within families, there may be pressure for higher levels of public services. This could increase the relative disadvantage of those with no families, if the level of services overall does not increase. It seems likely that spouses and in-household relatives (the latter mostly women) will continue to provide personal and domestic care at high levels to disabled elderly people, and that without substantial improvements in public domiciliary and home care services only people with access to this kind of informal support will be able to remain in the community at high levels of disability (Wenger 1992). Such improvements can be, but rarely are, achieved.

In the current climate of expressed commitment to "practical support" for carers will we see the development of sensitive and appropriate strategies of support for elderly spouses, as Wenger (1990) has advocated? Real support for the people giving most intensive care would mean that the current distribution of services, in which people in joint households hardly figure, would have to change. Unless people who live alone are to receive less this again suggests a need for an increase in public services. Alternatively we might see the continuance of the strategy observed by Pollitt et al. (1991) whereby professionals and relatives are able to turn a "blind eye" to the difficulties experienced because of elderly people's and other carers' declarations that they can manage. This is not meant to imply that such declarations are not to be respected at the time they are made, or that help should be forced on people who do not require it, but as one daughter who had cared with great difficulty and little help for a dying parent, observed after the event:

> I could have had a lot more help if I'd known . . . the district nurse came *once* and said "Are you happy to do what you're doing?" I said "I suppose so" so no one came again. (Seale 1990: 420)

Genuine practical support for family carers demands a more proactive approach from services. It also demands a willingness to support people who, although they may benefit greatly from help, would in any case continue to provide care for sick or disabled relatives even without support. However, a much more likely scenario seems to be that demographic and economic changes of the kind outlined will mean that there are more people with needs for care but fewer people with access to intensive family care; under new funding arrangements public resources will increasingly be targeted on those who would otherwise be admitted to residential care – mostly those without family support. Already there is evidence that rules being developed by social services departments for determining priorities will ensure a service only for people in danger of physical or emotional harm or liable to deteriorate if not supported. Under such a system, services will be provided only when resources permit to those whose "quality of life might be improved" but who are not seen to be at risk (Hoyes et al. 1992). Such priorities, whilst understandable, must mean that situations where a carer exists and does not express an intention to give up will be less likely to receive assistance. Hence the grounds for criticism that services operate by rewarding "failure to manage" by carers, will be intensified, and the risk will be increased that inter-

118

vention, when offered, will come too late to have any preventative effect. Finally, middle-aged women and older women and men will continue to bear an increasing share of the costs of caring, thus threatening the quality of family relationships by removing any element of choice about caring.

CHAPTER 6

Inheritance and financial transfer in families

Janet Finch

Introduction

It has long been recognized that, in a society based on the private ownership of property, inheritance is the key mechanism through which wealth and the privileges associated with it are kept within the control of one sector of the society (Engels 1884, Macfarlane 1978, Townsend 1979, Davidoff & Hall 1987). This happens because, except very unusually, it is the custom in such societies for property (of all types) to pass from one generation to the next within the same family.

Until the early 1970s it was only a small proportion of families for whom inheritance was likely to have any relevance, since most people possessed very little to transmit to subsequent generations apart from items of personal rather than monetary value. However, the spread of home ownership potentially changes all that. A house is a valuable asset and the rise of owner occupation from around one-third in 1960 to around two-thirds in the mid-1980s (*Social Trends* 1993) means that many more people will be in a position to pass on some wealth to their children and grandchildren. Indeed there is a sense in which this has been the explicit intention of recent governments in the UK, who have seen their twin aims of expanding private ownership of property and strengthening the family coming together through the mechanism of inheritance. The prime minister, John Major, has described his vision for the future as one in which he would want to see wealth "trickling down the generations".

There are many interesting questions that one can pose about the effects of this apparent extension of the relevance of inheritance to a wider range of people. In this chapter I shall focus on the question: what impact does inherited wealth have on the life-chances and life-styles of younger generations? Since I shall look at this question in relation to ordinary families, the types of families who have been drawn into the net of inheritance since the mid-1970s rather than those who have significant wealth, I use the term "wealth" very broadly here, to refer to any inherited capital assets. In "ordinary" families there is the potential for an inherited capital sum to make a significant difference to life-chances by enabling the beneficiaries, for example, to buy into the housing market for the first time, or to establish a small business, or perhaps to send their own children to private schools. How important is inherited wealth in shaping the lives of younger generations in families where the most significant asset in the estate is likely to be a house (or its value when translated into money)?

In discussing these questions I shall draw on findings from a study in which I have been involved of inheritance, property and family relationships, comparing it as appropriate with other research.[1] I shall use two types of data from this study. First, we have analyzed a randomly selected sample of 800 probated wills, from people who died in the years 1959, 1969, 1979 and 1989. Our reason for selecting these four sample years was to enable us to see whether there have been any changes in the pattern of bequeathing over that period of time when the rate of home ownership has been rising. Secondly, we have conducted in-depth interviews with 98 people about their personal experience of inheritance, and how these matters are handled in their own families. In some cases, we were able to interview several members of the same family.[2] This study population was selected theoretically rather than sampled statistically. Because of the focus of the study, the majority of interviewees were home owners, but within that we included people in a range of economic and family circumstances. Some were first generation home owners whilst others came from families who had owned their own homes for several generations.

Who inherits?

In looking at the impact of inheritance on the life-chances of younger generations, we need first to examine the issue of who does actually inherit. In the broader spectrum of families for whom inheritance is now an issue, are assets normally passed from parents to children and

121

thence onwards down the direct line of descent? Are other people included? How thinly are assets spread? The answers to these questions are important because they indicate how far inheritance remains a way of preserving wealth within those social groups who already have it, albeit now affecting a wider range of families than in the past.

In broad terms it seems that transmission to members of one's family remains the norm. In the 1970s the Diamond Report found that over 90 per cent of wealth transmitted through inheritance goes to relatives (Royal Commission on the Distribution of Income and Wealth 1977). In our own study, we found that 82 per cent of testators bequeathed to kin exclusively, and a further 14 per cent to a mixture of kin and nonkin. There was little change over our four sample years in the tendency to bequeath to kin exclusively.[3]

Within that overall picture of keeping assets in the family, which kin are favoured? Are assets passing from parent to child, and on further down the direct line of descent, or are they spread more widely? In general, passing down the direct line of descent does seem to be the norm, provided there is no surviving spouse. Leaving aside estates that pass to people in the same generation (primarily but not exclusively a surviving spouse) the testator's children are much more likely than any other group to figure as beneficiaries. For example, in a study based in Scotland in the 1980s, Munro (1987) found that 43 per cent of the wealth was passing to spouses and 23 per cent to children, including stepchildren. Other relatives figured at a much lower level (Munro 1987: Table 8).

In our own work, we have looked at the likelihood of different beneficiaries appearing in the will, rather than attempt to estimate the comparative value of bequests.[4] Our data show that spouses are mentioned in 37 per cent of wills and children in 36 per cent. Again, other categories of relative appear much less frequently. The most common (though not universal) pattern is that the surviving spouse inherits the main portion of the estate undivided, though children may receive specific bequests of personal items. In our sample spouses typically received either the total estate or the residue.[5] In the case of total estate bequests the spouse almost always inherited 100 per cent of the estate; where the estate had been divided into gifts plus residue, spouses received on average 93 per cent of the residue. Thus typically children receive the total estate, or the residue, only if there is no surviving spouse. However, if this is the case, children are much the most likely beneficiaries for these types of bequests.

There is a general tendency therefore to concentrate on the nuclear family in inheritance matters and, in the absence of a surviving spouse, this means that children generally are treated as having the major claim. However, what this actually means to an individual child will depend on whether the estate is divided between several children or passed intact to a single individual. There are some limitations here in the conclusions that one can draw from bequests in wills, since a bequest to just one child may mean either that the testator has only one surviving child, or that other children exist but are receiving nothing. Our own data show that 39 per cent of wills that mention children name only one child and 61 per cent bequeath to more than one. Bequests to more than one child normally give to each child gifts that (as far as one can detect this from the wills) are roughly of equal value. It is difficult to estimate value precisely because often bequests to children include different specific personal items bequeathed to each child (for further detail see Finch & Wallis 1993, Finch et al. 1995).

Thus we find that it is more common than not to divide the estate between children, and this may well be very much the norm where the testator has more than one surviving child. What does this tell us about the impact of inheritance on the life-style and life-chances of children who are beneficiaries? This is a question with implications at the macro-level of the society as a whole, as well as for individuals, and has many historical resonances. The issue of whether estates are divided or not, and the effects of that upon the socio-economic structure of any society, is a matter that has been much debated in historical work on inheritance undertaken by social historians, anthropologists and historical demographers.

The principle of a single heir versus division of the estate has also been long debated publicly as, for example, Thirsk (1976) shows in her interesting discussion of English legal treatises and other writings of the sixteenth and seventeenth centuries. This debate arose from the fact that primogeniture (bequeathing the whole estate to the eldest son), less dominant in earlier historical periods, was gaining ground among the nobility in various parts of Europe during this period, though in England it was practised in a more extreme version than elsewhere. The English debate focused essentially on the position of younger sons, who quite commonly were completely disinherited. Some argued that this treatment was grossly inequitable, whilst others took the view that it was essential to political stability to have single heirs who would be the clear heads of their families and rulers of their estates (Thirsk 1976). In the early nineteenth century the issue was once again opened up as a consequence of changing practices. The new bourgeoisie of the early phase of industrialization were more likely to divide their wealth between a surviving spouse and their children, with daughters and sons both inheriting but typically receiving different types of gifts, than to practise straightforward primogeniture (Davidoff & Hall 1987).

This debate about equity of treatment for all children, versus the preservation of wealth in the hands of a minority, has contemporary parallels. Our evidence from wills, that children appear to be treated equally, is supported by our interview data where the principle of equal treatment of children is a strong theme. Indeed, as we have argued elsewhere, it can override other considerations even where it is clearly the case that one child has a closer relationship with the parent than another, including circumstances where one child has taken fuller responsibility for the parent's well-being (Finch & Wallis 1993). In some ways this is not surprising, given that more general evidence of parent–child relationships in adult life also suggests that equal treatment is seen as a fundamental of family life (Allatt & Yeandle 1986, Finch & Mason 1993).

Thus the principle of primogeniture would seem to be quite out of place in the context of the "ordinary families" who have formed the focus of our own study, and we really have found no trace of it in practice. The alternative approach – that of dividing the estate between surviving children on broadly equal terms – would seem to be firmly embedded as a cultural norm. This has interesting implications for the distribution of wealth, particularly in a situation where an increase in home ownership means that wealth derived from housing will be transmitted within a larger number of families. Now, as in the past, the custom of dividing an estate must mean that each individual derives smaller economic benefits than would be the case if wealth passes intact to a single individual.

If wealth is thus spread more thinly, it follows that the impact of inherited wealth on the life-style of each member of the younger generation will be more limited than it would have been in times when there was a single heir. In absolute terms, the impact of course will vary with the size of the estate. A proportion of a large estate may still be a sufficiently substantial sum to make a significant difference to the economic position of children who inherit. However, most estates are still not large, despite the inflation in house prices that occurred in the late 1980s and would have been reflected in the size of estates of home owners dying during that period. In 1989, the latest year of our wills sample, less than one-quarter of estates (21.5 per cent) exceeded £100,000. Three-quarters fell between £40,000 and £100,000.

If sums of this order are being divided between two or three children, the impact of the inherited capital on life-style and life-chances would be significant only if it were being bequeathed to individuals whose life circumstances were very modest at the time of inheriting. We have no means of knowing the circumstances of beneficiaries in our own wills study, but other research suggests that most beneficiaries are likely to already be fairly comfortably placed. In particular research by Hamnett et al. (1991) has shown that it remains the case now, as it has been in the past, that the overwhelming majority of people who inherit houses are already themselves home owners. Partly this is a consequence of the fact that home ownership is still concentrated in higher socio-economic groups. The analysis of Hamnett and his colleagues shows that households headed by someone in social class I or II are four times more likely to inherit as those whose head is classified as social class IV or V (Hamnett et al. 1991, see also Ch. 8). But it is also a question of when beneficiaries inherit – the issue to which I now turn.

When do beneficiaries inherit?

The question of when beneficiaries inherit is important because it affects the impact that inheritance is likely to have on their own life circumstances. The evidence that most people who inherit houses are themselves already home owners suggests that the potential impact of housing inheritance is reduced, in that people are receiving capital from this source when they themselves are already established in the housing market. Though inheritance may afford the opportunity to upgrade one's accommodation, in few cases does it appear to provide the opportunity to take the crucial first step.

What is true of housing inheritance is also true of inheritance more generally, for reasons that are straightforwardly demographic. Most people cannot expect to inherit from their own parents until they themselves are well into middle age because of the "unprecedented twentieth century revolution in longevity", which alters the structure of family life and social life by changing the circumstances under which people age (Riley 1985: 334). The effects of this in the British context have been spelled out in an important article by Anderson (1985). He shows that a combination of longer life expectancy and the age at which people bear children has served to alter substantially the average age of children at the death of their parents. Children born as late as 1891, in a family that was statistically typical, could expect both parents to be dead by the time the average child was aged 37. The corresponding figure for children born in 1921 was age 47. But for children born in 1946, in a statistically typical family, the children could expect to be aged 56 before both parents would be dead.

The effect of these demographic patterns on inheritance is extremely significant. It is clear that, for generations born since the Second World War, few can expect to inherit from parents until they themselves are contemplating retirement. Thus the potential for inheritance to affect life-chances in a significant way is substantially reduced by comparison with the past, though of course it may facilitate the beneficiaries' capacity to live comfortably in old age. Looked at in purely demographic terms therefore, in the late twentieth century inheritance can have a significant effect on the life-chances of younger generations only if resources "jump a generation" and pass straight to grandchildren, who would be at an age when an injection of capital might make a significant difference.

Is there any evidence that this is happening? Certainly the evidence suggests that it is rare for grandchildren to benefit directly from inheritance in any substantial way. Though grandchildren appear in wills, they were named in only 14 per cent of our sample. Of more significance, where they do appear they do not normally receive shares of the total estate or the residue. Only 16 per cent of wills that name grandchildren give them a share of these bequests; this represents just 2 per cent of all wills. This is in line with Munro's (1987) finding from Scottish wills that only 1 per cent of estates go to grandchildren. In our wills sample the most common bequest to grandchildren (71 per cent) is a cash gift, often on quite a modest scale. For wills probated in 1959, 1969 and 1979 the most common amount was £100. In 1989 this had risen to £1000, a significant increase but still not a sum of money large enough to make a difference to the grandchild's position in the housing market or to alter life circumstances in any significant way.

These data refer to first choice beneficiaries, but many wills provide also for the possibility that the first choice will predecease the testator. They therefore named grandchildren as substitutes rather than as first choice beneficiaries, though this occurs most frequently as a group bequest (to all my grandchildren) rather than to named individuals. Of wills that named substitutes, 22 per cent contained a group bequest to grandchildren, but only 5 per cent bequeathed to individually named grandchildren as substitutes. In circumstances where a person dies without a will grandchildren would also stand to inherit as substitutes; that is, if their own parent dies before the grandparent, the grandchildren are entitled to the share of the estate that would have passed to their own parent, had the parent still been alive (see Finch et al. 1995 for further discussion). Thus, as substitute beneficiaries, grandchildren do stand to inherit major portions of their estate directly. However, the likelihood in practice of estates' passing to grandchildren directly must be deemed remote, for the demographic reasons already mentioned. Increasing longevity means not only that people are likely to die at a more advanced age, but also that their own children will still be alive to inherit, except unusually. Thus, if grandchildren do benefit from inheritance, this must normally happen indirectly, that is, from assets that pass directly to the first generation descendant and thence are passed straight on to the next generation.

Jumping a generation?

Looked at as a matter of simple economic rationality, demography and family sentiment would seem to combine to create pressures for inherited wealth to "jump a generation"; that is for people who typically will inherit in late middle age to pass their inherited wealth straight to their own children, who should be able to use it to much greater effect to enhance their own life circumstances. Is there any evidence that, even though grandchildren do not normally inherit directly, "ordinary" families nonetheless are using inherited wealth in this strategic way?

Of its nature such evidence is much more difficult to glean than is evidence about who benefits directly through wills or via the intestacy laws. At this point I turn to our interview study, where we were able to ask people about the experience of inheritance in their own families, including questions about the more complex dimensions of what happens in reality. For the purpose of this discussion I have analyzed all references in these interviews to grandchildren inheriting from grandparents, either directly or indirectly. A total of 28 of our interviewees talked about this. They were drawn from across the full age range (the youngest was 18, the oldest 83); some of them talked about having received bequests from their own grandparents, some about bequests that have been promised to them, others about their intentions to bequeath to their own grandchildren.

In general what our interviewees told us confirms the patterns that I have identified from the wills study. Typically bequests from grandparent to grandchildren (whether talked about in retrospect or in prospect) were small gifts rather than major shares of the estate. Though certainly some interviewees saw cash gifts as appropriate (as the wills study indicates) they actually talked much more extensively about passing on items of personal property. These were usually items of jewellery or household ornaments, and what people talked about was the symbolic significance of such objects. For about half of this group of interviewees, these questions of symbolism dominated their discussion of bequests to grandchildren. The issue is well articulated by Simon Hilton, a single man in his early twenties whose grandmother had already identified objects to be given to each grandchild well before her death:[6]

> My gran's got a box full of stuff waiting for me when, when she pops off. . . . It goes back to when I was really young. You know, she asked all her grandchildren what they'd want when *she popped off*. And with me being smaller, there was these little pottery things – like little jugs and little cups and things like that – and I said "I'll have those". And she's remembered all this time, you know. She's popped them in a box. . . . She's got loads of silver spoons, loads of dolls from different parts of the country, and loads of coronation mugs, stuff like that. So they're all going to different grandchildren.

Simon discussed what he would receive in some detail and then was asked by the interviewer what he thought he would do with the items of pottery when he inherited them. He replied, "I'd never give them away. Because they aren't just jugs. They're part of my past."

So symbolic importance, rather than material value, is very much the dominant theme in relation to bequests to grandchildren. This is very different from the idea of using inheritance strategically so that major bequests jump a generation. Only six of our interviewees talked directly about the issue of inheritance jumping a generation, and all were lukewarm at best. All were hostile to the idea of inheritance passing directly to grandchildren, missing out the intervening generation. This was seen as the parental generation being cut out of a process that rightfully should involve them. But what of passing on wealth "indirectly"? Is it seen as appropriate for the parental generation, on receiving bequests from their own parents, then to pass them straight to their children who would derive more direct benefits from receipt of a capital sum? This type of thinking, though impeccably rational on economic grounds, is not reflected among our interviewees. No-one talks about passing on assets straight to their children. Our younger interviewees, who would be the potential recipients of such arrangements, do not appear to even speculate that their grandparents' death might bring them economic advantage. Our interviewees operate on a very different type of rationality, which can be understood if it is seen in context.

What our interviewees are saying to us about the grandchild generation is, in effect, that they should wait their turn. This is expressed in several different ways. For example there is a clear message in our interviews that no young person should receive a large sum of money before they can be guaranteed to spend it wisely. This is a view shared even by our youngest interviewees. For example Ian Lamb, aged 18 when we interviewed him, had in fact been left a sum of money (he thought that it was about £400) in his grandmother's will. He had expected to get access to it at 18, but when he reached that age his parents told him that he was not to be allowed to have it until he was 21 – a decision that he appeared to treat as entirely reasonable.

But the idea of grandchildren waiting their turn goes wider than simply letting them grow up before allowing them to have anything more than pocket money. It also implies that they should not expect to have access to significant amounts of "family money" until their own parents have died; the assets and the control should remain with the oldest living generation. That represents a taken for granted assumption in our whole set of interviews. However, to understand its full implications, we need to set alongside it another strong theme in the dynamics of families – that parents should continue to assist their children in adult life, financially as in other ways. This emerged as a prominent feature in our earlier study of family responsibilities and obligations (Finch & Mason 1991, 1993) and is certainly reflected among our interviewees in the inheritance study.

When we put together these two normative themes – that control of family assets should remain with the oldest living generation, and that parents should go on helping their children throughout adult life – we can see clearly why inheritance does not "jump a generation" either directly or indirectly. In the "ordinary" families whom we have studied, the oldest living generation expects not only to have assets under its own control, but also to use those assets as part of the *normal* process of parents helping their children. Inheriting money from one's own parents enhances one's capacity to give adult children financial assistance, but on a scale and at a time of one's own choosing. This seems to be the rationale on which our interviewees operated rather than seeing inherited wealth as assets to be used strategically by passing them straight to the next generation.

This point can best be illustrated by quoting in some detail from our interview with Eddie Giles. Eddie articulates these points in relation to his own situation more clearly than most interviewees, though undoubtedly the sentiments that he expresses are widely shared within our study population. Eddie was aged 37 when we interviewed him, married with two daughters aged 9 and 12. He worked as a plant operator in a large industrial complex, having served an apprenticeship as a fitter and turner and then worked in skilled manual jobs all his adult life. Eddie owned his own house with his wife Jackie, whom we also interviewed. In the following extract, Eddie describes a conversation that he and Jackie had recently with her parents, where his parents-in-law explicitly raised the question of whether they should bequeath their assets to Jackie and Eddie, or to their grandchildren.

> Eddie: They were asking us the other week. It's very difficult when someone says "What do you think we ought to do? Do you want us to leave our money to you or do you want us to leave it to the kids?" Now they asked us that the other week. . . . And it's a very difficult position to be put in really.
>
> Interviewer: Yes.
>
> Eddie: You know, you'd say "No. I want it all". You know. "Don't give our kids any. We want it all". Because if it did happen before they were really mature, I mean they could blow everything, couldn't they?
>
> Interviewer: Yes . . .

Eddie: I said "You can do things, like say they have to get it at a certain age, or maybe that they have to use it for a specific purpose". You can do all sorts of things in wills, can't you? "Or" I said, "you could leave it to your son and daughter and hope that they will do it fairly, you know, distribute the money that you will leave fairly down to the children".

Interviewer: Mmmm.

Eddie: But it was a very difficult position to be put in. Because we, me and Jackie, we have always planned to try and help them buy their houses, you know, when they first get married, and things like that. Now if we've been left it and we've still got the money, we'll be able to help them quite substantially.

In this interview Eddie makes it quite plain why the logic of jumping a generation is at odds with the ways in which family life normally operates. Even to raise the question creates great awkwardness: he keeps saying that it was a "very difficult position" to be put in. The awkwardness comes partly from the fact that it is difficult to argue that the money should go to himself rather than his children without appearing avaricious – a problem that he deals with by trying to suggest ways in which bequests to his children could be sensibly arranged.

But there is also a sense in which Eddie feels compromised by being called upon to justify the custom of passing assets to the next living generation – until that time, he had simply taken this for granted. His justification is partly pragmatic, concerning the need to ensure that children do not inherit at an age when they might squander the money ("if it did happen before they were really mature, I mean, they could blow everything"). But he also conveys a sense that he would feel cheated out of the opportunity to act as a "good parent" if the money had passed direct to his children. What he talks about is not the idea of receiving an inheritance and then passing it straight on. Rather he talks about plans that he and Jackie have already laid, in other ways, to ensure that they will be able to assist their children to buy houses and to set them up in married life ("if we've been left it . . . we'll be able to help them quite substantially"). Eddie treats the prospect of receiving an inheritance from his parents-in-law as enhancing their capacity to be good parents. It would go into the pot from which

131

he and his wife draw in their continuing parenting activities. However, this is a pot that they both reserve the right not only to control but also to use in other ways: "If we've been left it *and we've still got the money*, we'll be able to help them quite substantially".

Conclusion

The picture that emerges from this study of inheritance in "ordinary families" is that the effects of inherited wealth are extremely diffuse, when viewed from the perspective of individuals. Though normally kept within the family, wealth is spread evenly between children, with small amounts going to other people, including grandchildren. Apart from families where there is a pattern of only children in several generations, the net effect of this must be to give many people some money, but no-one a great deal. Dispersal of wealth rather than concentration is the norm.

The effects of inheritance are also diffuse in another sense. Typically beneficiaries inherit in late middle age, and therefore have long passed the time where inherited money could make a substantial difference to their life circumstances in the housing market, in employment, in enhancing educational opportunities. There is therefore no obvious way in which inherited wealth is reinvested, except possibly to enhance comforts in old age. It is apparently not passed on to the next descendent generation for their immediate use, either directly or indirectly. Some of it undoubtedly does get passed to the grandchild generation, but only some of it, and not immediately, and probably in a way that is not recognized as passing on inherited wealth explicitly. It simply becomes part of the resources that parents may chose to use to help their adult children at particular points in their lives.

So in ordinary families, where earlier generations would have had very little to bequeath, the new possibilities for the use of inheritance have not – as yet – developed a strategic dimension. People do not think in terms of conserving wealth intact and building it up to a substantial fortune (as was the case under the custom of primogeniture), nor do they seek to alter the balance of resources available to each generation. In a sense therefore John Major's metaphor of wealth trickling down the generations is apposite. But the trickle is not the kind of trickle that comes from a dripping tap, which flows from a single source to an identifiable exit. The more appropriate imagery is that of the mountain stream that, as it descends, divides and redivides, over rocks and underground, beginning from a single source but flowing through many exits, which could be traced only with great difficulty.

Looked at from the perspective of individuals therefore, the amount of money likely to be received through inheritance, and the point in the life-course where it comes, means that wealth obtained through inheritance plays little direct part in changing life-chances. What it does is to enable the recipients to give more assistance to their own children, though the scale and nature of this is unpredictable. In this sense the new possibilities afforded by inheritance seem to produce less significant effects in practice than many people suppose.

However, if one switches from a micro to a macro perspective, the picture is rather different. The way in which inheritance is used keeps assets well within the boundaries of the family directly descendent from the testator for the most part, even if it is spread quite thinly within those boundaries. Thus it can be used to maintain the collective position of such families within the socio-economic structure – to ensure that there is usually some resource that can be drawn on when needed, enabling parents to go on helping their children at strategic points. This may not amount to great wealth for any individual, but it does mean that some level of capital resource is available in those families where home ownership has become embedded and has resulted in wealth being passed on through inheritance. The spread of home ownership has meant that this will become progressively the experience of the majority of families, creating an ever clearer minority who have neither the ownership of their own property nor access to inherited wealth that results from property ownership in earlier generations. Hamnett et al. (1991) estimate that, on present levels of house ownership, in the future a minority of the population numbering between 10 per cent and 30 per cent will *not* inherit; the same people are also likely to fall into the minority who do not own property. Thus as government policies emphasize increasingly self-help and reliance on family resources rather than a publicly funded welfare state, the focus of researchers' interest will surely shift away from the advantages gained by those who have access to inheritance, and towards the disadvantages suffered by those who do not.

Notes

1. I would like to thank the ESRC for providing funding for the Inheritance Project (Grant No. 000232035). The research team comprised myself, Jennifer Mason and Judith Masson as research directors, plus Lynn Hayes and Lorraine Wallis as research associates. I would like to thank other members of the team for their contributions to the project on which this chapter draws, though they bear no responsibility for any errors of interpretation that it may contain.
2. The wills were sampled from the probate calendars for each of the relevant years, held at Somerset House. Half the sample came from people who had died in the south-east of England, the other half from the north-west. The interviews were mainly conducted with people living at the time in the north-west of England though in a few cases, where we were following up members of families, they lived elsewhere.
3. Patterns of bequeathing revealed in our wills sample are explored in depth in Finch et al. (1995) *Wills, inheritance and the family*, Oxford University Press.
4. Our approach to the analysis of wills differs from other studies in that we have looked at *all* beneficiaries, rather than concentrating on the "main" one. We have done this for two reasons. First, the focus of our project was on what wills can reveal about people's concepts of "family" and who should inherit; therefore we were interested in everyone who appears in wills. Secondly, we have reservations about whether it is possible to identify from wills who actually does receive the most valuable portion of the estate. The reasons for this are explained in note 5.
5. Bequests of the total estate occur in wills where no items are selected as specific bequests, but all the testator's assets (money, house, stocks and shares, personal possessions and so on) are treated collectively as constituting the estate. That estate is then bequeathed to one or more beneficiaries; if more than one, it will be divided in specified proportions. The alternative format for a will is gifts plus residue. That is, specific bequests are made (of money or of possessions) and what remains constitutes the residue that – like a total estate – is bequeathed to one or more beneficiaries. In the case of estates that take the form of gift plus residue one cannot be absolutely certain who receives the bequests of greatest value. Whilst in most cases it appears that the gifts are small by comparison with the residue, there are cases in which one cannot be certain whether, for example, gifts of items of jewellery might outweigh the value of the residue. It is for this reason that we have reservations about the concept of "main beneficiary" as used by some other researchers.
6. The names used in this chapter are pseudonyms.

CHAPTER 7

Housing inheritance in Britain: its scale, size and future

Chris Hamnett

The continuous labour of your life is to build the house of death.
(Montaigne)

Introduction: the inheritance scenario in the 1980s

Inheritance has been a fact of life for generations. Witness the Victorian melodramas regarding the "reading of the will". Inheritance was a key element in the work of novelists such as Trollope, Eliot and Galsworthy. The prospect of inheritance or disinheritance was a Damocles sword, shaping the fate of the upper and middle classes. The working classes did not figure much in the novels of inheritance, largely because they had little or nothing to inherit. Inheritance, like wealth, was concentrated in the hands of a small minority of the relatively well off (Harbury & Hichens 1979). Most wealth was transmitted intergenerationally rather than built up by the fruits of one's own labour (or that of others) (Harbury 1962).

Inheritance quietly went its own way, the province of probate specialists and the wills columns of the quality newspapers until the 1980s, when there was a sudden surge of interest in housing wealth and housing inheritance in the mass media and among politicians, financial analysts and commentators. *The Economist* (1988) in an editorial "Growing Rich Again" argued that:

> Britain's middle classes, so long demoralized and impoverished [*sic*], are about to grow rich again. Two main mechanisms are

changing the way money is distributed in Britain. One is inheritance; the other is tax reform. The generation of Britons now reaching retirement age was the first to put a big proportion of its savings into home ownership. Houses have proved a wonderful investment and those pensioners, often caricatured as poor, are really growing rich, but their riches are tied up in the roofs over their heads. Only when they die, bequeathing their property to their children, can this most popular form of British investment be cashed in. So the bequest, a staple of Victorian melodrama, is about to make a come-back.

Writing in the *Observer*, Neal Ascherson (1986) suggested:

Under the surface of London, there are strange tremors. Something is rising to the surface. . . . That something is middle class money. . . . The theory begins with something now familiar: the price of private housing in central London. Ever since about 1970, the value of this housing stock . . . has been rising steeply. . . . Until now there has been a habit of regarding these colossal values as "fairy money". . . . But cashing in time is coming. It's a matter of time and generations. . . . Now the older occupiers of "fairy money" houses and flats are beginning to die. The heirs do not need the property left to them, and will sell it. What this means is that in the next decade or so the upward mobile middle and professional classes of London will acquire staggering reserves of liquid cash.

The reason for this sudden interest in housing inheritance is straightforward and is based on two principal factors. First, the rapid expansion of post-war home ownership has meant that wealth ownership is now much more widely spread than ever before. In 1951 there were 3 million owners (31 per cent of households). By 1991 there were 15.4 million owner occupied dwellings (67 per cent of households). In the space of just 40 years Britain changed from a nation of private tenants to a nation of home owners. Secondly, the 1970s and 1980s were decades of massive house price inflation. From 1969 to 1989 national average house prices rose from £5,000 to £60,000 at current prices: an increase of 1,100 per cent. Not surprisingly this had a dramatic effect on personal wealth. The value of dwellings as a proportion of net personal wealth rose from 18 per cent in 1960 to 37 per cent in 1975 and 52 per cent in 1989 (aided in part by the sharp fall in the stock market in the early 1970s). Between 1970 and 1988 there was a sharp reduction in the share of personal wealth taken by the top 10 per cent of wealth owners and a considerable increase in the share of the top 50 per cent. The bottom 50 per cent of wealth owners (most of whom are not home owners) gained relatively little.

The dramatic increase in the level of housing wealth in Britain, combined with the realization that the ownership rates for the over 65s had risen sharply during the 1970s and 1980s and the rapid increase in the number of elderly households led to the view that Britain was about to see a rapid surge of housing inheritance. In 1951 there were 5.5 million people aged 65 and over (11 per cent of the population). By 1981 the number had risen to 8.5 million (15.5 per cent) and by 1991 it had risen to 9.9 million. The size of the elderly population is projected to remain static during the 1990s but the rates of home ownership among the 65+ age group have risen from 44 per cent in 1975 to 54 per cent in 1990, and it should rise to over 60 per cent by 2000 as those in middle age (who have higher rates of ownership) move into the older age groups. Thus a report on housing inheritance produced by merchant bank Morgan Grenfell (1987: 8) argued that:

> The effect of increased property ownership in the 25–40 age group during the fifties and sixties is now being reflected in high owner occupation rates for the retired population. Half of heads of households in the UK over 65 years of age are now owner-occupiers; this is likely to approach two-thirds by 2000. As a result there will be a large increase in property inheritance accruing to a majority of households over the coming years.

Saunders (1986) also declared that:

> With 60 per cent of households now in the owner occupied sector in Britain . . . not only is a majority of the population now in a position to accumulate such capital gains as may accrue through the housing market, but for the first time in human history, we are approaching the point where millions of working people stand at some time in their lives to inherit capital sums far in excess of anything they could hope to save through earnings from employment.

The prevailing view in the late 1980s was that, as Eden's property owning democracy came to fruition, Britain would become not just a nation of home owners but a nation of inheritors. As Nigel Lawson, Chancellor of the Exchequer, stated in a speech in 1988:

> We are about to become a nation of inheritors. Inheritance, which used to be the preserve of the few, will become a fact of life for the many. People will be inheriting houses, and stocks and shares.

Britain was perceived to be on the brink of a major social revolution that would lead to a wave of housing inheritance affecting a large proportion of society, particularly the middle classes whose parents had the foresight to buy good homes in the interwar years or in the 1950s and 1960s. The purpose of this chapter is to examine the evidence on housing inheritance, its scale and value, in an attempt to shed light on the validity of these assertions. It will be argued that while inheritance is an important phenomenon, most commentators in the 1980s fell into the trap of assuming that all home owners would leave their property to their beneficiaries and would not seek to extract any of the equity from the property prior to death. In fact, extraction of housing equity rose considerably in importance during the 1980s and some home owners now sell their home to pay for private residential care.The importance of equity extraction lies in the fact that the amount of equity tied up in housing is finite. It can be either transmitted via inheritance or extracted prior to death, but not both. Put simply, the greater the level of equity extraction, the less the amount available for inheritance. The more of one, the less of the other.

The following section examines the Inland Revenue figures on estates passing at death, and the basis of the data and their exclusions. This is followed by an analysis of the number, value and distribution of these estates, and the asset composition of estates. The chapter looks at the importance of housing inheritance within estates, and the changes in the number and value of estates with housing. The chapter then examines projections on future housing inheritance and compares these to figures recorded by the Inland Revenue. It also examines the importance of various forms of equity extraction, particularly the growth of residential care for elderly, and finally it assesses the future of housing inheritance.

The Inland Revenue statistics on estates passing at death

The basic source of information on the scale, value and asset composition of estates passing at death is produced annually by the Inland Revenue Service (IRS). Since 1968–9 the IRS have included figures on UK residential property as a separate category. This information is collected for the purposes of taxation rather than analysis of inheritance, and the figures are based on a stratified sample of applications by executors for grants of representation or probate for deceased persons' estates. This source has advantages and disadvantages. On the positive side, it is consistent and comprehensive in terms of the categories for which it collects data. As estates of over a certain minimum value require a grant of representation, a grant of probate or letters of administration before they can be legally administered or distributed to beneficiaries, evasion is limited and the figures are comprehensive. No probate, no inheritance. The size of the sample varies by age of the deceased and size of estate. For the under 45s 100 per cent of estates are sampled. For the over 45s, the proportion of estates sampled rises progressively from 2 per cent of estates up to £40,000, to 100 per cent of estates worth over £1 million.

The value of estates may be depressed by the transfer of assets prior to death to avoid inheritance tax, but this is more likely to result in a reduction in the value of assets rather than failure to enter the statistics at all. The cuts in inheritance taxation rates and the increase in thresholds since the early 1980s have reduced the incentives to avoid inheritance tax for all but a minority of wealthy individuals and few estates escape the Inland Revenue net. Until 1980, inheritance tax began on estates over £25,000 at a rate of 10 per cent, rising progressively to a peak of 75 per cent on slices of estate of over £2 million. In 1984 the top rate of tax was cut to 60 per cent and the system remained stable till 1989 when graduated taxes were replaced by a flat rate of 40 per cent over £110,000. This was subsequently raised to the current threshold of £150,000. As a result, the proportion of recorded estates liable for tax fell from 11.1 per cent in 1985–6 to 8.5 per cent in 1988–9 and the amount raised by tax remained stable at about £1 billion per year. This is only a tiny proportion (5 per cent) of the total value of estates.

The problems with the Inland Revenue statistics concern exclusions not avoidance. There are two major exclusions from the IRS statistics. First, joint property passing between spouses is exempt from tax and a formal account is not always submitted for property that is exempt. Secondly, orders made by the Administration of Estates (Small Payments) Act 1965 permit small estates containing certain assets up to a value of £1,500 (raised in 1984 to £5,000) to be dealt with without production of a grant. As many people, particularly tenants, have little in the way of assets, these two exclusions together account for the fact that the Inland Revenue statistics on "estates passing at death" average around 270,000 per annum or only 40 per cent of approximately 660,000 deaths annually.

This may seem a significant omission, but as the excluded estates are either small estates with assets under £5,000 or where joint property passes between spouses, the exclusions are unlikely to have a significant effect on housing inheritance as they do not involve a significant intergenerational transfer of assets. As the IRS (1986: 100) notes:

> The main assets which can be transferred without a grant of representation are National Savings, cash, some bank and building society accounts, consumer durables and insurance policies. Between 1976 and 10th May 1984, the amounts in any individual asset could not exceed £1,500 and, in practice, the estate would rarely exceed £10,000; for deaths on or after 11 May 1984, the upper limit per asset has been £5,000 with few estates above £25,000 administered under these provisions. An excluded estate can therefore include a dwelling only if it is owned jointly in such a way that the deceased's share passes automatically to the surviving joint owner.

Because it is now more common for property, particularly house property, to be owned jointly by a husband and wife rather than just by the husband, it is likely that there are now more excluded estates involving house property than there were in the 1960s and 1970s. This will delay but not eliminate entry of property into recorded statistics as surviving joint owners eventually die. The next section examines the evidence from the Inland Revenue statistics.

Trends in numbers of deaths and estates passing at death

The number of deaths fluctuates from year to year. Since the mid-1960s it has varied from 645,000 to 681,000 annually, but the long-term decline in mortality has meant that the number of people dying each year has fallen slightly since the late 1970s. The number of deaths in 1986–7 and 1987–8 was 645,000 compared to an average since the mid-1970s of 660,000. OPCS projections of number of deaths in future years do not suggest a significant increase. On the contrary, the number of deaths is projected to fall until 1995, and then slowly recover to 2015. The numbers of deaths should then increase as the post-war baby boom begins to die. The number of estates passing at death and the number of inheritances are thus very unlikely to rise between 1995 and 2015.

The Inland Revenue figures show that there has not been an increase in the number of estates recorded passing at death since the early 1960s. In 1963–4, the Inland Revenue recorded 316,000 estates passing at death. This fell to 267,400 in 1967–8 as a result of the Administration of Estates Act 1965 that raised the limit on the value of exempt assets from £100 to £1,500 and thereby reduced the number of grants of representation required.

The number of recorded estates during the 1980s averaged 275,000 per annum though it fell to 245,071 in 1985–6, 234,700 in 1987–8 and 249,233 in 1988–9. The fall reflects the raising of the small payment exemption limits from £1,500 to £5,000 in 1984, but it also reflects the decline in the number of deaths. There is thus no evidence of a rise in the number of recorded estates passing at death. Britain may become a nation of inheritors, but it is unlikely to happen for some years yet. Although perhaps 50,000 small estates have been removed from the IRS statistics by the rise in the exemption limits, the scale of inheritance in Britain has remained broadly stable for many years.

Not all recorded estates are available for inheritance by children and other beneficiaries. A substantial number of estates pass to surviving spouses even though the property is not jointly owned and thus exempt from the statistics. The scale of these transfers can be estimated from the Inland Revenue data on the marital status of the deceased.

In 1986–7 48 per cent of male estates belonged to married males (65,576 out of a total of 135,603 male estates). Some 16 per cent of female estates involved married females (21,463 out of a total of 135,344). Thus, a total of 87,039 or 32 per cent of the 271,947 estates involved married persons. The average since 1989 is 33 per cent. While some of the property may well pass to children or other beneficiaries, it is likely that in the majority of cases, the bulk of the estate will pass to the surviving spouse. This will reduce the number of estates available for non-spouse or intergenerational transfers by one-third to approximately 180,000 per year.

The number of beneficiaries

The figures given above are for the number of estates passing at death. The number of main beneficiaries is far larger. Analysis of a survey of beneficiaries carried out by National Opinion Poll (NOP) for Hamnett & Williams (1993) found that the mean number of major beneficiaries per estate is three. Taking the figure of 180,000 non-spouse estates, this suggests a total of 550,000 individual non-spouse beneficiaries per annum. This is approximately 1.2 per cent of adult individuals and 2.4 per cent of households (assuming individual inheritances occur in separate households).This may not seem a large proportion but over a 10 year period, 12 per cent of adult individuals and 24 per cent of all households could inherit.

The value and distribution of estates passing at death

Although the number of estates passing at death has not increased since the mid-1970s, the value of inheritance has risen dramatically, primarily as a result of inflation but also as a result of the growth of home ownership. The total net value of estates rose from £1.9 billion in 1968–9 to £20.2 billion in 1989–90: an increase of 950 per cent. The average value of estates rose from to £7,100 to £72,800 over the same period. The average number of main beneficiaries per estate is 3.0, which suggests that each beneficiary would have inherited just over £24,000 on average in 1989–90.

The average value of estates is useful as an aggregate measure of change over time, but it is very misleading as a measure of the distribution of estates by size because the distribution is very negatively skewed. In other words there are many small estates and few large ones. The average is inflated by the small number of large estates. Looking first at the number of estates in each category in 1987–8,

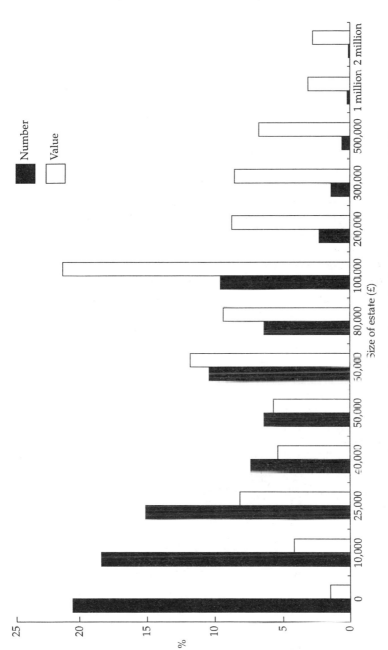

Figure 7.1 Distribution of estates by number and value, by size band, 1987–8 (%).

Figure 7.1 shows that the largest number (21 per cent) of estates were worth under £10,000 closely followed by the £10,000–25,000 (19 per cent) and the £25,000–40,000 (15 per cent) categories. No less than 55 per cent of estates were worth under £40,000 and 69 per cent were worth under £60,000. Only 33,464 estates (14 per cent) were worth over £100,000, and only 10,743 (5 per cent) were worth over £200,000. Just 470 estates were worth over £1 million.

The distribution of estates by value makes the point even more clearly. The 40 per cent of estates worth under £25,000 account for only 7 per cent of the total value of estates, and the 69 per cent worth under £60,000 account for only 26 per cent of total value. Conversely, the 31 per cent of estates worth over £60,000 account for 74 per cent of the total value, and the 0.9 per cent of estates worth over £500,000 account for no less than 13 per cent of total value. The distribution of estates by number and value is shown in Figure 7.1. It can be seen that while the great majority of estates are relatively small, the lion's share of estate by value is concentrated in a relatively small number of large estates. Dividing average estate size by the number of beneficiaries suggests that the 21 per cent of beneficiaries of estates of under £10,000 would have inherited only £1,500 on average and 40 per cent of beneficiaries would have inherited £6,000 or less in 1987–8. These are small sums but as the average size of estate increases, so does the average per beneficiary. Thus, the average value of the 10 per cent of estates worth £100,000–200,000 was £136,000 and beneficiaries would have inherited £45,000 on average.

The asset composition of estates passing at death

The relative importance of different assets

Housing is now by far the most important single component of inheritance by value. In 1988–9 it accounted for 47 per cent of the total capital value of estates, more than double the value of cash, bank and other interest bearing deposits (21 per cent) and stocks and shares including government and municipal securities (18 per cent). No other assets were worth over 5 per cent of the total (Table 7.1). The importance of housing has increased very considerably since the late 1960s when it accounted for only 24 per cent of the total net capital value. The high share in 1988–9 reflects the late 1980s housing boom and the 1987 stock market slump. The proportion will fall back once again as a result of the current slump in the home ownership market.

Table 7.1   Asset composition of estates passing at death, 1988–9.

	Value of estate (£ million)	Capital value (%)
UK residential buildings	8,439	7.1
Cash, including bank and interest bearing accounts	3,740	20.9
UK company securities	2,330	13.1
UK government and municipal securities	867	4.8
Insurance policies	617	3.4
Other personalty	552	3.1
Household goods	404	2.3
UK land	414	2.3
Trade assets and partnerships	208	1.2
Other UK buildings	147	0.8
Loans and mortgages	97	0.5
Overseas and foreign securities	53	0.3
Foreign immovables	26	0.2
	17,908	100

Source: Inland Revenue, 1993

The categorization of estates by asset composition

The importance of housing and other assets within estates varies by size of the estate and it is possible to split estates into three broad categories by asset composition. Small estates are those under £25,000, medium estates are those between £25,000 and £100,000 and large estates are those over £100,000. Each type of estate has a different pattern of assets (Figure 7.2). The three different types of estates can be described as small cash estates, medium estates dominated by house property and large estates dominated by stocks and shares and land.

In small estates under £10,000, cash, bank and other interest bearing deposits are the single largest asset at 55 per cent, followed by insurance policies (12 per cent) and government and municipal securities (12 per cent) such as national savings certificates and premium bonds. Small estates generally have few stocks and shares or residential property. As estate size increases the importance of cash, insurance policies and government securities falls, and in medium sized estates worth £25,000–100,000 housing accounts for 50–60 per cent of total assets. Its importance then steadily declines with size of estate as other assets such as stocks and shares increase in importance.

In large estates the relative importance of stocks and shares rises from 14 per cent in estates worth £100,000–200,000 to 48 per cent in

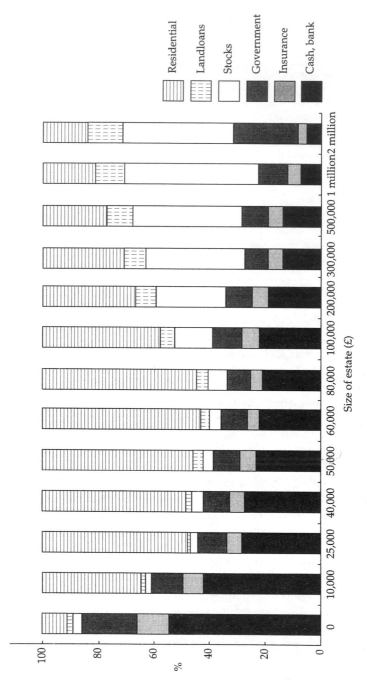

Figure 7.2 Asset composition of estates passing at death by size of estate, 1987–8.

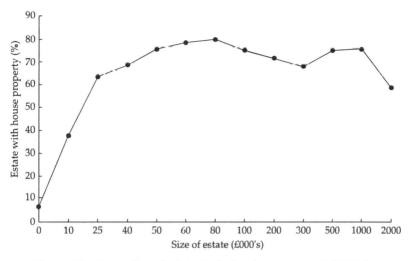

Figure 7.3 Proportion of estates including house property, 1987–8.

estates worth £1 million–2 million. The importance of land and other buildings also rises from 1 per cent of estates worth under £10,000 to 14 per cent of estates worth over £2 million.

Although housing is included in only about 55 per cent of estates this figure is depressed by the relatively large number of small estates under £25,000 that do not contain house property. Figure 7.3 shows that in estates over £25,000, the proportion including housing ranges from 60 to 80 per cent. This proportion has risen very considerably since the late 1960s. In the following sections we examine the scale and value of housing inheritance given its considerable importance.

Inland Revenue data on the scale of housing inheritance

The prophets of an "inheritance economy" suggest that the scale of housing inheritance is likely to grow rapidly in the future. Moreover because home ownership and the proportion of older home owners has been growing rapidly since the 1950s, there is an implication that the scale of housing inheritance should have increased since the mid-1970s. But Inland Revenue statistics show no evidence for a long-term increase in the number of "estates passing at death" including housing. On the contrary, the number of estates containing house property

147

Table 7.2 Number and value of estates passing at death.

	Number of estates with UK dwellings	Total no. estates (£ million)	% of total	Value of housing (£ million)	Total value (£ million)	%
1968-9	125,085	271,238	46.1	465	1,923	24.2
1969-70	149,592	287,239	52.1	501	1,948	25.7
1970-71	142,473	267,718	53.2	530	1,967	26.9
1971-2	149,052	288,796	51.6	638	2,275	28.0
1980-8	143,343	294,841	48.6	3,057	6,883	44.4
1981-2	147,894	295,236	50.1	3,280	7,628	43.0
1982-3	143,980	288,199	50.0	3,383	8,211	41.2
1983-4	148,800	296,890	50.1	3,683	9,195	40.0
1984-5	147,717	273,762	53.9	4,163	10,372	40.1
1985-6	137,486	245,071	56.1	4,567	11,482	39.8
1986-7	149,265	270,947	55.1	5,398	12,738	42.2
1987-8	125,532	234,688	53.5	6,020	14,310	42.1
1988-9	140,561	249,233	56.4	8,439	17,320	48.7
1989-90	154,225	276,412	55.8	9,460	20,121	47.0

Source: Inland Revenue Statistics, various years.

has been broadly stable through the 1970s and 1980s at around 145,000 per annum (Table 7.2).

The number of estates containing residential property has grown slowly and erratically, from 125,000 in 1968–9 to 154,000 in 1989–90: an increase of only 23 per cent. But the 1968–9 figure is abnormally low and may reflect some initial under recording. If 1969–70 is taken as the base year, the number of estates has scarcely grown at all and has merely fluctuated between 125,000 and 154,000 estates averaging about 145,000. These figures clearly contradict the claims made by the pundits for the growth of housing inheritance.The picture to date has been one of stability rather than rapid growth.

Housing inheritance and spouse beneficiaries

The figures in Table 7.2 include all estates containing house property, but some of these will pass to surviving spouses even though they do not own the property jointly. It is thus important to exclude these properties as they are not available for inheritance as commonly defined. The published Inland Revenue data on assets by sex, age and marital status do not identify house property as a separate category. They do, however, identify a category of "net land and buildings" that is broadly comparable and used as a surrogate. In 1989–90 about 64,000 estates with land and buildings belonged to married persons. This proportion (41 per cent) is broadly stable from year to year and reduces the 154,225 estates including houses to just over 90,000: far fewer than commonly supposed.

The value and distribution of housing assets in estates

What has clearly changed is the proportion of estates containing house property. This rose from 46 per cent in 1968–9 to 56.4 per cent in 1988–9. The value of housing inheritance has also risen dramatically: from £465 million in 1968–9 to £9.46 billion in 1989–90. This is an increase of almost 2,000 per cent in just over 20 years. The value of inheritance overall also rose from £1.92 billion to £20.12 billion, an increase of 950 per cent. Non-housing inheritance increased in value by only 632 per cent. The value of housing inheritance therefore rose twice as fast as inheritance in general and by 3.2 times the value of non-housing assets. The increase in the total value of inheritance since the mid-1970s owes a great deal to the increase in the value of housing assets. As housing makes up around 47 per cent of the total value of estates, it has been the driving force behind the increase in the value of estates since the mid-1970s.

As the number of estates containing housing has risen only slightly since 1968–9, the growth in the value of housing inheritance is almost entirely the result of house price inflation. This is simply shown if we compare the figures for 1968–9 and 1987–8. In both years the number of estates containing house property was 125,000. But the value of the housing assets increased from £465 million in 1968–9 to £14.3 billion in 1987–8. This has important implications for the future value of housing inheritance and inheritance in general. The sharp fall in average house prices from 1989 to 1992 will soon be reflected in a sharp decline in the value of house inheritance or, at best, a sharp fall in the rate of increase. The delay is occasioned by the fact that the Inland Revenue statistics run about three years behind owing to the inevitable delay in collecting information. The value of house property in estates should also be reduced by around 40 per cent to take account of property passing to spouses. In 1989–90 this would reduce the value of house property from £9.46 billion to £5.35 billion: much less than commonly thought.

The distribution of house property in estates

The distribution of estates by size containing housing differs from the distribution of all estates. Although few estates worth under £25,000 contain house property, house property is then strongly represented in the middle value estates from £25,000–100,000. The proportion of estates with house property is less than the proportion of all estates in the larger size bands. The distribution by value of all estates, and house property is very similar, however.

Table 7.3 shows that the number of estates containing house property are greatest in the small to medium wealth bands of £10,000–200,000. These bands contain a remarkable 91 per cent of estates including house property. The concentration by value is slightly less but these estates still include 81 per cent of total residential value. The concentration by value is at its peak in estates valued at £60,000–200,000. But the distribution of house property is more evenly distributed than that of other assets.

Table 7.3   Residential property passing at death, 1987–8.

Value estate (£)	Number	%	Cumulative %	Amount (£ million)	%	Cumulative %
0	2,897	2.31	2.31	24.8	0.41	0.41
10,000	16,850	13.42	15.73	274.3	4.56	4.97
25,000	23,406	18.64	34.38	630.9	10.48	15.45
40,000	12,389	9.87	44.24	420.7	6.99	22.44
50,000	11,886	9.47	53.71	464.4	7.71	30.15
60,000	19,875	15.83	69.54	1,013.3	16.83	46.98
80,000	12,825	10.22	79.76	753.1	12.51	59.49
100,000	17,545	13.98	93.74	1,307.8	21.72	81.22
200,000	4,024	3.20	96.94	413.9	6.87	88.09
300,000	2,322	1.85	98.79	342.4	5.69	93.78
500,000	1,164	0.93	99.72	224.6	3.73	97.51
1 million	280	0.22	99.94	87.4	1.45	98.96
2 million	70	0.05	100	62.5	1.04	100
Total	125,533		100	6,020.1	100	

Source: Inland Revenue, 1990.

A nation of inheritors? Who inherits house property?

Peter Saunders (1986) suggested that millions of working people will inherit property. Other commentators have been less sanguine. Both Morgan Grenfell (1987) and *The Economist* (1988) suggested that housing inheritance would tend to accrue to existing home owners, particularly to the middle classes. Evidence from two large national surveys of beneficiaries carried out in 1989 and 1991 (Hamnett 1991, Hamnett et al. 1991, Hamnett & Williams 1993) shows that the great majority (*c.* 80 per cent) of beneficiaries have, in fact, been existing home owners. They also show that, while the majority of beneficiaries are in the intermediate and junior non-manual and skilled manual occupational groups, the incidence of inheritance is far higher among the professional and managerial socio-economic groups than it is among other groups (Table 7.4). Hamnett (1991) has shown that this is a result of the parental class and tenure backgrounds of beneficiaries rather than beneficiary characteristics. The current distribution of housing inheritances reflects the characteristics of home owners a generation ago when home ownership was much more restricted to the middle classes than it is in the mid-1990s. It can be argued as a corollary to this, that the distribution of housing inheritance will widen considerably between 1995 and 2025 as the current generation of home owners leave property to their beneficiaries.

Table 7.4 Distribution of housing inheritance by class.

	A	B	C1	C2	D	E	Total
Inheritors (N)	84	342	356	323	145	76	1,326
% distribution	6	26	27	24	11	6	100
Total sample	323	1,415	2,306	3,134	2,005	1,461	10,644
% incidence	26	24	15	10	7	5	12

Source: NOP survey for Hamnett et al. 1991

Projections of the future scale of housing inheritance

The projection of the scale of housing inheritance has been fairly simple to date. All the projections start by applying age specific death rate to home ownership rates by age group to produce estimates of the number of dying home owners each year. These figures are then reduced to allow for the proportion of two-person households in the

151

age group where the survivor is assumed to take ownership and continues to live in the property. This method can be used to produce retrospective estimates of the scale of housing inheritance that can be compared to recorded Inland Revenue figures for previous years.

Several projections have been made of the likely future scale and value of housing inheritance. The first was by Morgan Grenfell (1987). Their methodology was not entirely clear,but they estimated a total of 155,000 cases in 1986 rising to 160,000 per annum by 1990, 178,000 by 1995 and 202,000 by the year 2000 (Morgan Grenfell 1993). In their 1993 projection the figures were revised downwards to 119,000 cases in 1986 rising to 128,000 in 1991, 180,000 in 1996 and 200,000 in 2001. The reason for this downwards revision of the earlier figures is unclear as the methodology remains the same. It may be an attempt to bring them into line with Inland Revenue figures for non-spouse transfers that are far lower than Morgan Grenfell's initial estimates.

The second projection (Hamnett et al. 1991) was more detailed and explicit about the methodology but arrived at similar figures. We projected a figure of 168,000 finally dissolving owner occupied households per annum in the five year period 1986–91, rising to 188,000 in 1991–6, 207,000 in 1996–2001, 227,000 in 2001–6 and 343,000 by 2026–31. This is double the current level, and given that there are three main beneficiaries per estate on average, this suggests that by 2036, 2 per cent of the adult population and 4 per cent of households could stand to benefit from housing inheritance every year other things being equal (Table 7.5).

Lloyds Bank estimates (James 1993) are based on estimated death rates among single person owner occupied households. Their estimates are much lower than either of the above estimates and suggest 133,000 transfers in 1991, 139,000 in 1996 rising to 153,000 in 2001.

The first three projections support the views of those who suggest that Britain is becoming a nation of inheritors. But the validity of the projections are dependent on the validity of their assumptions and

Table 7.5 Comparisons of different projected levels of housing inheritance: number of non-spouse transfers (000s).

	1986	1990	1995	2000	2005	2010
Morgan Grenfell (1987)	155	160	178	202	–	
Hamnett et al. (1991)	–	168	188	207	227	246
Morgan Grenfell (1993)	111	128	180	200	220	235
Lloyds Bank (James 1993)	–	133	139	153	–	–

some of these are very questionable, particularly the view that house inheritance is a direct, unmediated, outcome of home ownership rates of the dying population. It will be argued that there are strong reasons for thinking that projected increases will not occur, and that some of the equity tied up in housing will leak out prior to death. For this reason, I consider that the Lloyd's Bank projections that suggest a level of only 153,000 transfers per annum by 2000 – some 50,000 a year below that of the other projections – may be more realistic. The number of cases of house inheritance is likely to increase only relatively slowly. Britain is unlikely to become a nation of inheritors, now or in the future.

Why has the scale of housing inheritance not increased?

We have seen that the number of estates containing house property between 1969 and 1990 has been broadly stable at about 145,000 per annum. This raises two major questions. First, why has there been no increase in the number of recorded estates containing house property given the rapid growth of post-war home ownership? Secondly, is the number of estates with house property likely to increase in the future? Several reasons can be put forward for the very limited increase to date, some of which are far more likely than others.

First, it can be argued that the Inland Revenue are under-recording the true number of estates containing house property. This is unlikely for reasons already set out. Secondly, it can be argued that the number of estates with houses has been reduced by tax avoidance measures such as gifting prior to death or establishing trusts. But this is unlikely to occur on a significant scale. Thirdly, changes in the gender relations of home ownership and a diminution in the number of sole male owners have led to an increase in the proportion of jointly owned properties passing automatically to the surviving spouse and reduced the number of properties entering into house inheritance statistics. This is extremely likely, but is difficult to quantify and will delay the release of property only until the death of the surviving joint owner. The time lag is unlikely to be more than 10 or 15 years at the very most.

The fourth reason is that the great expansion of home ownership in the post-war period has not yet percolated down into inheritance. There was only a limited growth of home ownership between 1939 and the early 1950s, and the majority of new post-war home owners are still alive. For example, a person who bought a house in 1960 aged 30 will be only 64 in 1994. This is undoubtedly very important and it does suggest that, in the absence of other factors, the number of housing inheritances will increase very rapidly between 1995 and 2025 as the home owners who bought in the 1950s, 1960s and 1970s gradually die off. It is worth reiterating here that the size of the elderly population and the size of the owner occupied sector has greatly increased since the mid-1960s and the proportion of home owners in the over 65s has risen from 44 per cent in 1974 to 54 per cent in 1990 and is likely to reach 60 per cent by 2000. But home ownership has been rising rapidly since the 1950s, and it was expected that the growing number of older home owners would have begun to percolate through into inheritance statistics.

None of the reasons considered above adequately explain the stability in the number of housing inheritances since the mid-1970s. To do so, two other factors need to be taken into account. These factors also suggest that levels of housing inheritance in the future may be far less than the simple projections would indicate: first, a growing number of elderly owners may be passing on their houses to their children prior to death in order to avoid paying for residential or nursing home care; and secondly, a growing number of elderly home owners are using the capital from their house, either to pay for residential care or to increase income as part of an equity release scheme. These factors are considered in detail below.

In the past elderly home owners had little option but to leave their property to beneficiaries. This is no longer true. Since the mid-1980s there has been a rapid expansion of private residential care for the elderly and of a variety of equity extraction schemes that enable elderly owners to exchange housing equity for income. There was a marked increase in both the number and variety of equity release schemes on offer to elderly home owners during the 1980s and in the number of elderly home owners taking up such schemes. The main types of schemes are mortgage annuities, investment bonds, rolled up interest loans and reversions. The characteristics of these schemes and the value of the equity involved are noted by Mullings & Hamnett (1992). We estimate that the number of equity extraction schemes is unlikely to increase significantly until the mid-1990s and it may double by the end of the decade to 10,000 per annum. This is not large, but it will depress growth of housing inheritance in the future.

The growth of private residential care for older people

The number of older persons in residential care in England and Wales has risen dramatically since the mid-1970s: from 143,000 in 1975 to 232,000 in 1988. All the increase has taken place in private residential care. The numbers of older persons in this sector increased from 19,000 in 1975 to 30,000 in 1980 and 102,000 in 1988. From 1980 to 1988 the number of persons in private homes rose 242 per cent, and from 1970 to 1988 the increase was over 450 per cent.

The number in local authority homes fell slightly from 110,000 in 1980 to 104,00 in 1988 and are likely to fall further as cash limited local authorities dispose of their homes to the private sector. The number of older persons in voluntary sector homes remained stable at some 26,000. The number of private nursing home places in the UK also increased rapidly from 37,000 in 1986 to 129,000 in 1991. Taking the UK as a whole, Laing and Buisson estimate the number of private residential and nursing home places in 1991 was 296,400 compared to 54,000 voluntary places and 120,000 local authority places. The 1980s have, in effect been characterized by privatization of residential care for the elderly. This care has to be paid for and it eats into housing equity (Hamnett & Mullings 1992b).

Private residential care is expensive. Laing and Buisson estimate that in 1991 average weekly nursing home fees ranged from £272 in northern England to £350 in the Home Counties and £434 in Greater London. The national average is about £300. Residential home fees are somewhat less but averaged about £250 per week. Costs have risen rapidly as a result of the high labour inputs and interest servicing. Given that 54 per cent of retired single persons (the group most likely to enter care) in the UK in 1990 had a gross weekly income of under £80, 69 per cent under £100 and 85 per cent under £150, it is very clear that the overwhelming majority of elderly persons cannot afford private care out of income. Laing and Buisson estimate that only 15 per cent of older people are able to pay for residential care and only 9 per cent are able to pay for nursing care out of income (McKay 1992).

Under current arrangements, government income support is available to pay care costs for those with assets of less than £8,000. Over this level, individuals or their families have to meet the full costs of private sector care. In the public sector individuals with assets of over £8,000 have 25p per week deducted for every £100 of assets they possess over the limit but the effect is much the same. It is likely to necessitate sale of the house in the majority of cases.

Although there is no direct evidence, there is clearly an incentive for older people likely to go into care to transfer their assets to their family to ensure that they are not eaten away by care costs. Although this may not be very common, there is no doubt that many older home owners are forced to sell their homes to pay for care. The average length of stay in care homes is approximately 2.5 years. This suggests an average turnover of residents of about 40 per cent. There are 470,000 nursing and residential places in total. This suggests 190,000 new entrants a year on average. Even a conservative estimate of 25 per cent turnover would indicate 125,000 entrants a year. The proportion of these who are home owners is not known with certainty, but if the tenure background of residents reflects the tenure composition of the elderly population as a whole some 44 per cent or 55,000 may be home owners.

On the assumption that two-thirds of residents are forced to sell their homes to pay for care, about 36,000 older home owners sell their homes each year. The actual figure could be higher, depending on the turnover rate and the proportion who have to sell. Holmans (1991) has estimated that 30,000 older owner occupied households were dissolved in 1990 through moves to live with relatives or into care. This figure would account for the difference between the projected number of properties inherited (168,000, 1986–91) and the numbers recorded by the Inland Revenue (145,000).

The NHS and Community Care Act 1990 that came into force fully in 1993 replaces automatic income support for residential care by a cash-limited sum allocated by local authorities for various forms of care provision. Because residential care is expensive relative to other forms of care, local authorities may allocate less money to residential care in the future. If owners wish to enter a residential home it may be necessary to sell their own home to pay.This may increase the number of houses that are sold in future. This is likely to partly offset increases in the number of older home owners and reduce the number of properties available for inheritance.

Conclusion

The rapid expansion of post-war home ownership combined with the rapid rise in house prices in the 1970s and 1980s led to the sudden realization that a large number of older home owners now owned

156

considerable housing assets. This led to frequent suggestions that Britain is set to become a nation of inheritors. These suggestions appear to be supported by the projections made of future levels of housing inheritance. But an examination of the Inland Revenue data shows that, rather surprisingly, there was no increase in the number of recorded estates passing at death that contain house property. The number has been remarkably stable since the mid-1970s and there is a shortfall of some 20,000–30,000 between projected "releases" in 1986–90 and the number of cases recorded by the Inland Revenue. When the estates of married persons are excluded from the Inland Revenue statistics (some 40 per cent of cases), the shortfall is even more dramatic. This poses considerable problems for the proponents of the nation of inheritors. Even though the value of housing inheritance has rapidly increased between 1968 and 1989, this is entirely a product of house price inflation.

The projections assume that the principal factor that influences the scale of housing inheritance is the level of home ownership among the older population. This has steadily increased since the 1980s and is set to increase further as high home ownership levels among the 30–55 year olds work through to older households. But the scale of housing inheritance is not just a result of ownership levels among the elderly. There are a variety of factors that may reduce or eliminate home equity prior to death. The significance of these other factors is clearly shown by the fact that the number of estates containing house property has not increased since the mid-1970s on the basis of the IRS statistics. This evidence is counter to the suggestion of steadily rising home ownership among the elderly population. The projections overestimate the current number of housing inheritances by 20,000–30,000 per annum.

Although the Inland Revenue statistics are problematic because of their exclusions (particularly joint property passing between spouses), and the possibility of transfer of assets prior to death, it is clear that the number of property inheritances recorded has not increased. A number of possibilities were suggested to account for this. They included an increase in numbers of joint property passing to spouses, the growth of inheritance tax avoidance (which is very unlikely), and a timelag effect before the growth of post-war home ownership percolates into inheritances. This is very likely and will have had some effect, but it would still be expected that some increase in the number of estates containing house property would have occurred.

It was argued that there has been a secular increase in the scale and volume of equity extraction prior to death, and that more older owners were likely to transfer their properties prior to death either to pay for residential care or, in some cases, to avoid payment. This is likely, but impossible to document. What is certain is that there has been a remarkable expansion of residential care for older people during the 1980s, and given the cost of such care, it is likely that many (but not all) residents have had to sell their houses to pay for the costs of care.

It is estimated that some 36,000 homes a year may be sold to pay for care, and that a further 2,000 per year may be lost to inheritance via equity extraction schemes. Also an unknown number of houses may be transferred by elderly owners to their children prior to residential care. These figures suggest that the number of houses actually passed on for inheritance is likely to increase only relatively slowly, at least until 2005. We are likely to see an increase in the scale of housing inheritance in the twenty-first century, but it is unlikely to reach the levels suggested by some projections as they simply assume that older home owners remain owners until they die and that the property is then transferred to beneficiaries. Such unmediated projections must be treated with considerable caution. The notion of a vast wave of housing inheritances in the 1990s is utterly improbable.

CHAPTER 8

Intergenerational relations in the labour market: the attitudes of employers and older workers

Philip Taylor and Alan Walker

Introduction

Intergenerational relations and solidarities are embedded in the labour market and, during the twentieth century, social policy has played a critical role in formalizing these relationships. Retirement emerged as a mechanism for rejuvenating the workforce and, in effect, represents a form of institutionalized generational succession. Much of the impetus behind the development of retirement was provided by the economic, medical and managerial theories of the late nineteenth and early twentieth centuries concerning the differences in industrial efficiency between younger and older workers (Graebner 1980). The most famous of these was F. W. Taylor's (1947) theory of scientific management. These theories tended to portray older workers as inefficient burdens. Although such theories were subsequently discredited scientifically, they have helped to construct prejudices that still exert an influence in the labour market (see below).

The purpose of this chapter is to present a preliminary examination of the issue of intergenerational relations in employment by means of data collected from a national sample of major UK employers and a smaller local sample of older workers. Our analysis is preliminary because the survey was not designed specifically to investigate this issue and, therefore, further research is required to pursue this vital but unexplored area. By way of background we begin by discussing the position of older workers in the UK labour market. This is followed by an outline of the samples and the research design. We then discuss the issue of intergenerational relations, first from the position of older workers, and secondly, from the position of employers, drawing parallels and identifying differences between the attitudes of older workers and employers.

An ageing workforce

At present two opposing trends, an ageing workforce and an increasing incidence of early exit from the labour force, are taking place in the UK and other advanced industrial societies (Kohli et al. 1991). The structure of the British labour force is undergoing a significant change with fewer young people entering the labour market. Between 1985 and 1989 the number of 16–19 year olds fell by 14 per cent (1.5 million school leavers). Between 1985 and 2001 it is predicted that the number of 16–19 year olds will fall by 21 per cent (2.5 million). Yet, at the same time, life expectancy has been increasing and in 1995 stands at 77.7 years for women and 71.9 years for men.

However, these demographic changes come against a background of a long-term trend towards earlier and earlier labour force exit among older people. The UK has experienced a decline in the employment of older men since the 1950s. This accelerated in the 1970s and 1980s and, as Table 8.1 shows, resulted in just over three-quarters of men aged 55–59, just over half of men aged 60–64 and less than one-tenth of men aged 65 and over being economically active in 1994.

The participation of women in the labour force has tended to increase slightly since the 1970s (Walker 1984) though, looking at the cross-sectional series shown in Table 8.1, it is important to bear in mind that the cohort effect of increased labour force participation of women in the post-war period is likely to coincide with many of the same factors influencing male participation in later life. Once the cohort effect of the post-war rise in female economic activity is disentangled from the cross-sectional picture shown in Table 8.1, a similar trend has occurred among older women, although it is less steep than the male one (Guillemard 1993).

The growth of early exit among British older workers is primarily the result of demand-side factors, particularly the recessions of the 1970s and early 1980s (Walker 1985, Trinder 1990). In fact it has been argued that "early retirement" or withdrawal from the labour market brought about by an increase in unemployment is better understood as a form of unemployment than as a form of retirement (Casey &

160

Table 8.1 Labour force participation of older men and women in Britain, 1951–93.

Age	1951	1961	1971	1975	1981	1985	1990	1993	1994
Men									
55–9	95.0	97.1	95.3	93.0	89.4	82.6	81.5	75.7	76.1
60–64	87.7	91.0	86.6	82.3	69.3	55.4	54.4	52.4	51.2
65+	31.1	25.0	23.5	19.2	10.3	8.5	8.7	7.2	7.5
Women									
55–9	29.1	39.2	50.9	52.4	53.4	52.2	55.0	53.2	55.7
60–64	14.1	19.7	28.8	28.6	23.3	18.9	22.7	24.3	25.6
65+	4.1	4.6	6.3	4.9	3.7	3.0	3.4	3.5	3.2

Sources: 1951–71 Census of Population for England and Wales and for Scotland; 1975–94 Department of Employment, *Gazette* (various); UK Labour Force Survey.

Laczko 1989). It coincided with a period of simultaneous contraction of full-time employment and historic high points in the numbers entering the labour force. Moreover when tackling the problem of unemployment young people were given higher priority by government than older ones. In fact during the post-war period older workers have been viewed by policy-makers as a labour reserve whose employment prospects rested on the supply of young recruits. Thus three separate phases may be distinguished in the fortunes of older workers. Immediately after the Second World War, when labour was scarce, older workers were officially urged not to retire and "sink into premature old age", but to work a little longer and, therefore, have "a happier and healthier old age" (Phillipson 1982: 33). A special government committee was established to encourage older workers to remain in the labour market. At the same time medical research began to show that retirement had detrimental effects and a "breakdown" theory of retirement was formulated.

As the supply of younger people increased, as immigration grew, and as greater numbers of women entered the labour market, these special measures receded. By the 1970s a dramatic turnaround had occurred in the attitudes of policy-makers and the general public towards older workers, with the main driving force behind this change being the upward spiral of unemployment. In 1976 the Trades Union Congress (TUC) passed a motion calling for a lowering of the retirement age for men to 60, partly in order to ease youth unemployment. Then, in 1977, intergenerational solidarity became a part of official labour market policy for the first time when the Job Release

Scheme (JRS) was introduced. It is true that the Redundancy Payment Act 1965 encouraged the shedding of older workers in preference to younger ones because of the age premium and industrial tribunals have "confirmed that it is acceptable for an employer to choose a worker nearer retirement age in preference to a younger employee" (Laczko & Phillipson 1990: 91), but the JRS represented the most explicit policy of generational substitution yet seen on the statute book. The scheme was introduced, as a temporary measure and on a limited basis, specifically to alleviate unemployment among younger workers by providing allowances for older people to take early retirement and be replaced by younger ones. It was extended by the Conservative government in 1981. The scheme reached its peak, along with unemployment, in 1984–5 when 90,000 older people were receiving allowances. In addition, from 1981 unemployed men aged 60–64 were awarded the then higher rate of supplementary benefit (now income support) if they agreed to withdraw from the unemployment register – a further means of encouraging older workers to leave the labour market. Moreover, older people were discouraged from seeking work by Job Centre staff and also experienced considerable discrimination from employers (Walker 1984, 1985).

Thus, in this context, the pressures on older workers, through the policies of employers, unions and government, were generally in the direction of exclusion from the labour force in preference for younger workers. It is not surprising therefore that such messages were internalized by some older workers. For example Walker (1985) gives examples of unemployed steel workers in their sixties who thought that their withdrawal from the labour market would leave a job vacancy for a younger person:

> . . . the fact that there were so many young people out of work and I thought I'd done a life-time's work and might as well leave it for the younger ones.

> It was more or less: no jobs available and I thought, "I've had a good run, give somebody else a chance". There are lots of others with young ones to bring up. It's a greedy world.

Similar expressions of intergenerational solidarity or sacrifice were reported in earlier research on early retirement (McGoldrick & Cooper 1980: 860).

The third phase began in the late 1980s when influential voices began to warn of a "demographic timebomb" in the mid-1990s when, it was predicted, there would be a shortage of up to 1 million younger labour market entrants (National Economic Development Office NEDO 1989). This prompted a series of policy measures to try to encourage older people to remain in or to re-enter the labour force. These include the 50 plus Job Start Allowance Scheme, whereby an older person received an extra amount on top of the wage or salary paid by the employer (the scheme was abandoned in February 1991 because of its low take-up) and the abolition of the earnings rule that penalized people who worked beyond pension age.

The government's "Getting-On" campaign is intended to educate employers about the benefits of employing older people. However, reflecting the government's desire for an unfettered labour market, legislation to outlaw age discrimination in employment is not favoured. In addition protection under unfair dismissal legislation does not apply after the state pension age. In the face of only limited efforts to improve the prospects of older people there is evidence that more blatant forms of age discrimination persist, such as the targeting of redundancies on older workers.

The status of early labour force exit as a key feature of government policy to control the labour supply since the 1970s means that its role is central to any debate about relations between the generations. Yet there is little up-to-date evidence on older workers' attitudes and the attitudes of employers towards the distribution of employment according to age. For example, we know little about older workers' views on work and retirement, how they view themselves in relation to younger workers and what they consider to be their place in the labour market. In addition, little is known about older workers' views on different retirement options such as partial retirement and greater flexibility in the age of retirement (Walker 1982). Similarly we know little about how employers view the issue of the relationship between age and the labour market. How much do they value older workers as against younger ones? Moreover there is no research on the impact of government initiatives in this area on employers' policies towards older workers.

Surveys of employers and older workers

In order to examine the relationship between age and the labour market we conducted a study between 1989 and 1992 of older workers' attitudes towards work and retirement and employers' policies and attitudes towards older workers. This research was funded by the Economic and Social Research Council (ESRC) under its second Ageing Initiative. The sample of older workers comprised a subgroup of a representative sample of 1,000 households in Sheffield drawn from the electoral register under an ESRC funded study of socio-political consciousness carried out in 1986. Detailed labour market histories and a range of factual and attitudinal data were collected from informants. For the purposes of this study older people in the age ranges 47–62 (men) and 45–57 (women) at the time of the original survey were re-interviewed. There were some 194 informants in these age ranges at the time of the original survey.

A total of 134 men and women were reinterviewed. Table 8.2 gives the number of respondents by their current employment status. The approximate mean age of the respondents was 57 years.

Table 8.2 Respondents by current employment status.

Employed	76
Self-employed	7
Unemployed	8
Early retired	16
Retired	7
Sick/disabled	8
Home maker	12

Questions that focused on older people's attitudes towards younger people were included in a mainly qualitative survey of the labour market experiences of this group of older people. Respondents were asked a range of questions about experiences of working and seeking work, covering job search, perceived barriers to an individual obtaining work, the extent of and reasons for job changing in later working life, the nature of such changes and the perceived attitudes of managers to the deployment of older workers, education and training, age as a criterion for recruitment and commitment to paid employment.

The survey of employers was divided into two stages. The first consisted of a postal survey of 500 large employers (those with more than 500 employees) covering a range of industries except agriculture, which was deliberately excluded. This sought information on company policy towards older workers: for example the extent of policies to recruit, retain or retire older workers and attitudes towards older workers. The second stage of the research consisted of in-depth interviews with 100 of these employers chosen to reflect the range of company policy towards older workers from the very positive to the very negative. This survey of company policies produced a considerable amount of data on the relationship between older and younger employees at the workplace that complement the data collected from the earlier survey of older workers.

Attitudes of older people

We asked older men and women about their perceptions and experiences of employers' attitudes towards older and younger workers. They believed that employers would see several advantages in employing younger people including the fact that they may be fitter, more attractive, have more working years ahead of them, be more trainable and be more adaptable to change than older people. It was also felt that younger people would often be considered more acceptable by employers because of their paper qualifications and experience with computers and new technology. New technology was frequently mentioned as an area in which younger people would have the advantage unless older persons had kept themselves up to date with technological advances. Some respondents felt that younger people were cheaper to employ although a minority view was that older people were cheaper to employ. The perceived views of employers are summed up by the responses of these selected respondents:

> Bit of a liability, sickness, slower, train them and it won't be for very long. If they've got skills want jobs you can't offer them, a higher job when you can't offer them one. They also jump above younger people. Don't think older people can take on computers as easy.

> My employer appreciates my experience as I've been in this trade all my life. Older workers have a more settled outlook and probably work for less money.

> Don't know, they're not interested in people over a certain age. There's a lot of emphasis on qualifications now, pieces of paper to do the job.

For many jobs I think 40 would be too old these days unless you'd kept yourself up to date with technology.

A number of respondents felt that there had been a recent change in employers' policy and attitudes towards the older worker. A few employers, we were told, had instituted early retirement schemes but had reversed this policy after finding that too many high quality staff were leaving to be replaced by younger, and in the opinion of our respondents, inferior staff. Older people considered themselves to be much more reliable than younger people, better timekeepers, more settled, more hard working and more concerned to do a good job. In addition, older workers considered that experience of working life was now being recognized by employers. Trinder (1990) also found that some employers had regretted making redundant so many older people during the recession of the early 1980s. These are some examples:

We are thought of as part of the fixtures and fittings. Old broilers we are called. But they know we are good workers not spending 20 minutes in toilets and being off ill for days on end.

I think they do now. They didn't at one time. It's altering now. They've been forced in to it. Got to have experience in some jobs that take years to actually learn with safety.

Probably see older workers as more reliable, especially with women. Younger ones leave to have a family.

Older staff can go on training courses at any time the same as young ones. They are very keen on training and they look after you pretty well.

On the other hand, among the non-employed workers several people felt that the best jobs were open only to younger people; while jobs for older people were more likely to be part-time and poorly paid. For example, one woman when asked whether she thought that there had been a recent improvement in the employment prospects of older people made the following statement:

I still think they want younger people. Older people, their jobs are often part-time and poorly paid. My daughter's friend earns more than my husband.

Among those people we interviewed, many thought that employers had misconceptions about how older and younger workers would relate together and about the productivity of younger compared to older workers. Stereotypical views about older workers were, according to our respondents, commonplace. In the words of two people:

I was an accounts clerk up to being made redundant and I'd rather do that to cleaning but I couldn't get another office job. I was told, at 49, for an office job they were looking for 18 to 30 year olds to blend in with existing staff. You weren't with it to fit in with younger staff. In my present job, cleaning, you are thought of as a good workhorse, reliable, honest etc. and it's appreciated. But in an office, men seem to think older women wouldn't get on with young ones which is not true.

I've never been idle and they'd probably get more work out of me than someone younger but I don't think employers think that. You can't even get as far as the interview stage.

According to the older people, these attitudes resulted in company policies that targeted younger workers at the expense of older workers. For example, there was a feeling that employers used the government's Youth Training Scheme (YTS) to obtain workers cheaply. On the other hand older people were needed for their skills and experience:

They want them [older workers] for their experience and skills. These days they seem to give youngsters six months training and send them out knowing next to nothing.

As I see it in my company, engineering, I look for a good apprenticeship. It never fails to produce sound engineering knowledge. These skills are lacking in youngsters today.

Because the very young ones offer them cheap labour. These YTS schemes and Job Centre schemes are all on the cheap.

167

Older people in our survey often held negative attitudes towards younger managers. They considered that younger employers and managers were particularly likely to discriminate against the older applicant or employee. In the words of two respondents:

> If it's a younger one doing the interviewing they definitely discriminate against the older applicant.

> A higher management team came in. All about 40. Said I'd be made redundant. I threatened them with court proceedings and in the end they said the job was redundant not me at 52. We went from fifteen of us in the same status down to just six in three years. Some were re-deployed but they wanted me to go out of Sheffield but wouldn't say where. I was utterly disgusted with the whole set-up.

Attitudes towards younger workers

As noted earlier, there is some previous research evidence that suggests that older people may be put under considerable pressure to retire early or accept redundancy and this sometimes entails reference to a duty to make way for younger people. Therefore we asked respondents whether employers should give younger people the first chance in recruitment. While we found some support for the view that younger people should take priority there was equal support for the view that employees should be selected on their ability to do the job. Some respondents felt that age should not be considered as a factor when making recruitment decisions while some thought that the older person had been given their chance and should now make way for the young. However, some older people felt that, where decisions about redundancy had to be made, it should be the younger people who would go first because they were less hard working and took more time off while others thought that many young people did not want to work and were not prepared to look hard for employment. Others considered that the crucial issue was how close the older person was to the pension age: with regard to those people nearest to retirement age younger people should be given the first chance, but for people in their fifties opportunities between young and old should be equal. Some thought that the state pension age should be lowered to give young people a chance and to reduce unemployment. The following are examples of what some respondents said on younger versus older workers:

It should be equal opportunity for everyone. If they're capable they should get the job simply on merit.

Think they prefer to take on young ones and train them for their future workforce. Young ones need a job. Lots of older married women have husbands to support them and they can be unreliable, having time off when children are ill.

If I'd got kids now I'd sooner they had the job than me. They lose confidence if they haven't got a job.

Other respondents considered that, as younger people were already given considerable support through training schemes,[1] older people should not need to make way as well. Similarly a view expressed by some older people concerned the relative chances of older and younger people finding work. Respondents questioned why, when younger people had better prospects of finding work, they should receive most help. In the words of one respondent: "A young person can try elsewhere. Yes, they've more chances of finding jobs."

Finally, some older people were aware of what is only just beginning to dawn on many employers: older workers have a critical role to play, often in wholly informal ways, in the training of young people. This includes specific on-the-job training (standing next to Nellie) and more general initiation into organizational culture in which older employees act as the repositories of the "collective memory". Thus, by removing older people from the workforce employers lose the only people with the skills to train the young workforce. In the words of one respondent:

You have to give young ones a chance but not at the expense of older workers. They've got rid of older people who could have been training young ones.

Attitudes towards retirement

When asked how they would feel if offered the option of taking early retirement in the near future views were mixed. Some respondents were keen to retire early while others thought that they would consider it carefully. Some would take it to spend more time with their spouse while others thought they could easily occupy their time in leisure pursuits. Others thought that they would accept retirement and take another part-time job to supplement their income. Job changes and job stress were given as reasons why early retirement would be considered. For example one man was so distressed about his situation as a headteacher that he said he would seriously consider taking early retirement if it were offered despite a substantial loss of income. One woman considered that she might be better off financially if early retired as, being a widow, she paid a substantial amount of her income in tax. Here are two examples:

> I'd consider it seriously. I've had enough under the present climate. The speed of the changes disillusions people. It would very much reduce my standard of living in financial terms.

> If the money is to my advantage I'd take it because as it is they stop so much tax as a widow I don't bring home much at all.

Early retirement was viewed negatively by others. This was often linked to income although many stated that they enjoyed their work and it was an important part of their life. In the words of two respondents:

> It wouldn't benefit me at all. If they offered me a lot of money I'd refuse. It's no good to me. I've years of work in me yet.

> I've got to work until I'm 65 as a condition of me getting a mortgage to be in this house. I couldn't afford to retire.

Employed but not self-employed respondents were asked if they would have to give up work at a certain age or whether they would be allowed to stay on in some capacity. Forty-three respondents stated that they would have to stop work at a certain age. This was usually the state pension age although some older women noted that their companies' policies had changed such that they could now stay beyond 60. A male civil servant stated that, at his grade, he was required to retire at 60. Twenty-nine people thought that they would be allowed to stay on, the rest were not sure. Of those thinking that they would stay on, the majority thought that it would be in the same job although three stated that this would be on a part-time basis.

We also asked respondents, if when they had to give up their present job, whether or not they would try and get another one. Twenty said that they would while forty-five said they would not. The rest were undecided. The results indicate that, for a majority, there was a desire to leave employment at state pension age. In fact there was often relief at thought of retirement. For some people this attitude was linked to poor health. For others, retirement was seen as a time for leisure activities and a time to spend with partner and family. It appears that measures aimed at encouraging this group to remain in the workforce would be a waste of effort for this group.

> I'll have had enough by then. My arthritis isn't going to improve with age, I doubt I'd be able to work longer.

> I'd like to go at 58 I think, my husband will be ready for retiring by then.

For others there was a feeling that they had done their bit and deserved their retirement. Moreover one man we interviewed had taken early retirement because he wanted to give a younger person a chance: "It's only fair. Elderly people have had their chance. I took early retirement [Job Release Scheme] because of it."

However, as well as a positive attitude towards retirement we found that a significant number of older people wanted to remain in work as long as possible. Many respondents did not want to retire because they enjoyed their jobs, while others preferred to remain in employment for financial reasons such as keeping up mortgage repayments and a lack of pension provision. The financially insecure included those people living alone, who were usually women. As noted by Walker (1982), it is women who face the most hardship in retirement because they are more likely than men to be disadvantaged in the labour market, particularly with regard to occupational pensions, and they tend to live longer. In the words of two women we interviewed:

> I don't have a choice. I'll have to keep on working as long as I possibly can.

> I'll have no works pension so I'd have to do something.

We asked those stating that they would try to get another job what they would be looking for and why. Some respondents thought that they might do voluntary work. For many the work they would want to do would be paid part-time work although others needed a full-time job for financial reasons. Meeting people, relieving boredom and getting out of the house were given as reasons for wanting to continue to work. In the words of one woman we interviewed:

> Not so many hours. Perhaps two a day. I couldn't be at home all day. I'd be bored. I'd look for a shop assistant's job or even cleaning. I wouldn't mind that because I'd need an interest in something and a bit of money is always useful. I'd be bored at home. I need an outside contact.

For others working after retirement was not so much a case of what they would want to do but rather who would employ them because of their age. Based on their own previous experiences of unemployment there was a feeling that efforts at finding another job would be unsuccessful. There was also evidence of job downgrading in later working life for some people who, following redundancy, are able to find only work that provides them with a much reduced income.

These results indicate that, according to the older workers themselves, their re-employment prospects are poor. To the extent that older workers believe that they would not get a job elsewhere they are in effect forced into taking and then become trapped in low skill, low responsibility and, therefore, low paid employment. In the words of three people:

> I wouldn't get another job if I left and I need the money, so can't think of leaving. I was an accounts clerk up to being made redundant and I'd rather do that to cleaning but couldn't get another office job.

> At my age you have to accept anything. I would like to carry on working.

> I put 30 year's service in for my firm as a service engineer and I got nothing, but miners and British Steel got anything from 20–30 thousand pounds for 24 years. I got four thousand pounds for 30 years. I couldn't retire on that. Glad to be working now but not earning anywhere near what I was before.

Flexible and partial retirement

We found considerable support among older people for policies such as phased retirement and greater flexibility in the age of retirement. A large majority of respondents favoured phased retirement while almost half favoured flexibility in the age at which an individual could claim their state pension. The freedom to choose when one retired was thought of as being important. Several respondents stated that they would be very interested in working until aged 70 or beyond while others wanted to retire at or around the age of 60. Health was frequently mentioned when talking about retirement. Some mentioned that those who had retired earlier looked healthier while others thought that it was work that kept them in good health. Some talked about staying in jobs that they could no longer cope with because they could not afford to give up work while others in good health felt that they would like to work as long as their health would allow. In the words of a few respondents:

Very interested. Well, some are ready for retirement but like me I can't bear to think of being bored. The social side is very important to me. We meet up and go out together regularly. I'd miss that side of things.

I like to work. Since my husband died I live for my work I like going out each day. Being on my own I need the job and the money.

In my case yes, as my husband is younger than me I would not get a pension until he retires, so I would like to work until after 65.

Similarly views on partial retirement were generally positive. A period of gradual easing into retirement was favoured by the majority of respondents although a minority felt that partial retirement would take away full-time jobs that could be taken up by younger people. A reduction in the male state pension age was preferred by some respondents as a solution to the problem of large scale unemployment. A small minority of respondents worked for firms or had partners working for firms where variants of partial retirement schemes were in operation. Some of the early retired we spoke to had experienced partial retirement programmes and were equally enthusiastic.

173

These are some examples of what respondents said:

> I had always worked. When I first stopped I had to see the doctor. It was done too quickly. I felt isolated and old.

> The firm I work at, if you have been there 25 years you go on to a period of run down, working four days a week for so long, then three, then two and finally one day a week. It's a good idea. It would be hard to just stop work.

> We had appraisal talks and they suggested cutting to three days a week. After 39 years of service. To get used to the idea of not working at all. That worked very well to our mutual benefit. To break me in gently from working flat out to doing nothing.

Attitudes of employers

There was a remarkable similarity between the responses of the older workers and the employers we interviewed to questions regarding the relative utility of younger and older workers. Employers tended to value older people more for their experience and stability than their skills, whereas younger people were valued more for their skills, particularly in connection with new technology. For example some employers, mindful of the fact that older staff were likely to stay with the organization longer than younger staff, were trying to increase the age ranges represented within their organizations in order to create a more stable workforce. In one company it was stated that older people were important as "uncle" or "aunt" figures but it was felt that there were positions not suitable for older people. In the words of a few personnel managers:

> I think that the only area which is starting to emerge is potentially the computer knowledge and skills and computer aptitude where there is now a generation of school leavers coming through who have substantial keyboard skills, computer skills, knowledge of various software computer programmes and everything else, which I think it's difficult for the next generation but one up to actually acquire in quite the same way. Not I think in many ways that we couldn't.

In another area we were having great problems bringing in school leavers into our technical laboratories in chemical analysis. And there, the problem is that all these youngsters come in, but they want a career, they want to go to the top. Now what we wanted was some stable people who were perhaps older, happy to have a job.

Well, we wanted to firstly increase the age profile to bring a bit more stability and experience in their experience that people had had as property accounts clerks a number of years ago, and were happy to come back now the children had become school age or what have you, rather than having younger people who, I have to watch what I say, we were spending a lot of money training on, and then they were going on somewhere else, and using those skills somewhere else instead of staying with us.

Younger people were also often considered more vibrant and energetic and cheaper to employ and one employer suggested that the media images of older people might be responsible for this. However, even in what might be described as relatively "young" industries there were jobs in which, according to some employers, experience was coming to be increasingly valued. In the words of one manager:

Then of course, you see sports activities much more on television. Tennis, athletics, and you hear of people being past it at thirty. "Good heavens, Jimmy Connors comes out as a veteran almost, at thirty – whatever he is – seven or something." Therefore young people must psychologically start thinking that they're old, forty years olds are old. And especially if they haven't been brought up with older people.

But I mean that's one way that things are changing in our industry. Experience is beginning to be respected, and business knowledge is beginning to be respected, because there are an awful lot of young people coming into the computer industry who are brilliant on the technical side, go off and set up on their own and then fall flat on their faces because they haven't got the business side of it right. So now it is more respectable to have been around a few years.

Contrary to stereotypes concerning inflexibility, some companies employed older people in jobs that involved considerable travel and periods away from home. Such jobs included engineers moving between different locations around the world and construction workers moving between sites. Older people were also seen as reliable and stable and having a stronger work ethic whereas younger people were seen as less reliable and not likely to stay with the firm for long. Older workers were valued by some service sector employers because their client group tended to be older and, it was felt, preferred to be helped by people closer to their own age. This was the case in, for example, department stores and homes for older people. The opinion of older workers held by many employers is summed up by this quote from a personnel manager:

Well they have a different attitude. They most certainly do. Whereas you know, if one of the young people have a headache or something they take a day off work whereas you know, older people wouldn't dream of that. I mean I've, from experience in retail, that was far more the case. You know, the old sales assistants I mean they would be there you know, on death's door almost because they were so loyal they would hate to let anyone down, whereas the youngsters, their attendance records – it was always the young people I was having to pull up because of their absence.

Other employers felt that older people were suitable for non-career jobs that a younger person would not want to consider. Some employers also stated that many school leavers lacked basic literacy and numeracy skills, which the company could not teach them, but which older people did not lack. Other employers felt that having a mixture of ages was important. There is no doubt, however, that some companies continue to foster a youth orientated culture. The view of some employers was that people could work in such a high pressure environment for a finite period of time before becoming "burnt-out". Elsewhere jobs had clearly defined career paths. For example other personnel managers felt that it would be a waste of a considerable investment if the opportunities for advancement were not available to a younger person. Accordingly efforts were made to clear the career paths of younger people. For example one personnel manager we spoke to stated the company had "a policy of trying to bring young people forward" and, in another company, the view of one manager was that "young people" in his words "were much easier to order around, tell them to do things my way, whereas more experienced people would want to be left to get on with the job themselves". In the words of some other managers:

> The manager will not take senior people in. He brings in school leavers and develops them. They're all trained and developed and they get their qualifications and they stay and the whole department's like that. He's like a father. He's quite firm at times. But it's for their own good and it works.

> These [older] people aren't going anywhere and these [younger] people can't get through. You then get to a dilemma, well what do you do? Are you prepared to waste all the money, effort and time you put in training these young people and let them go to another organization so that other organization gets the benefit? Or do you try to make gaps in the organization and that's what we did around 1980.

> What I would see as an ideal situation, is that the working life, the paid employment life, the essential paid employment period should be within that particular range that would start from the school leaving of about 16 and finish up somewhere at about 55. But from there on people who were "retiring", yes they may go to another paid employment, they may set themselves up as consultants and do that sort of thing.

Similarly in other organizations "trainee" and "graduate" posts were reserved for younger people and some others wanted to recruit younger people to mould them in the ways of the particular organization. In some private sector companies the main issue was economics: employers were recognizing the benefits of employing older people but younger people were cheaper. In the words of a few personnel managers:

> I wouldn't employ somebody over 50 in a job where they were on equal terms with a lot of very young people, so I wouldn't have a 50 year old in our trainee intake.

177

I think in the financial services industry, there is a culture of young people doing high performance jobs, and we have seen quite a number of staff who have asked or we have felt in both the companies and their interest to retire in their fifties, and so we see that quite often. The venture capital industry is quite a tough industry.

I think in the professions which this [accounting] is, there is a kind of youth culture and it's driven by this very rapid rise to the pinnacle of the career which is the partnership.

It is, I think, in the current market, perhaps people are much more aware that the quality and the expertise of people coming in at an older age group, is more valuable than maybe, taking on a school leaver. But again, you're coming up against the economics of a school leaver is cheaper.

A related point made by one respondent was that youth orientated companies would employ younger managers who would show hostility towards older people. A personnel manager from a major supermarket chain felt that, at the end of the 1980s, concern about a lack of school leavers led to the development of policies aimed at attracting young people, to the detriment of looking at other parts of that labour pool. The reasoning behind this strategy may be explained in part by the view of another personnel manager who stated that she had noticed that many of the employing managers she met were young people and that recruitment agencies tended to be staffed by younger people. She felt that this situation would be likely to lead to discrimination against older people. However, a personnel manager from a bank stated that he would "like to think, that if they [a recruitment agency] believed there was somebody aged 55 who was as vibrant and energetic as a 30 year old, that they would give us a ring and say 'well look this person's outside the specification but you really ought to see them'." In the words of a few other employers:

We're an industry that rewards young people and if you're suggesting that there will be, the market place will have an over supply of older people and a shortage of supply of younger people, we don't believe that this is the situation from our information. But if it were then I think that we are an industry that does very well reward young people for their efforts at an early age. So I think we wouldn't probably have the pressures that some other industries might have.

I think as often as not the intolerance of youth in the sense of if there are perhaps some people in middle management positions or whatever who are comparatively young they do perceive the older people as not having the energy, the dynamic approach, being set in their ways, unchangeable or whatever.

It's been difficult to try and recruit at the moment because we don't need anybody. I mean this is the big problem isn't it. It can't only be us. At the moment, certainly from the bottom end, the school leaver end, I mean there's no problem and that's always been very much our policy has been a bottom up and through the ranks sort of situation. Only very recently have we started to move away from that slightly to start recruiting people from an experience point of view.

On the other hand a few personnel managers stated that, in their organizations, team working was very important and teams were made up of a mixture of experienced and less inexperienced individuals. For example in advertising, it was argued, it was important to employ younger and older people so that adverts would be produced by people who could relate to the age group in question. Elsewhere this was not always the case. In the words of three personnel managers:

It's all very well taking the young high fliers, but they are flying high and tend to leave the nest pretty quickly, so yoo they might he able to move your business very rapidly in terms of being very innovative, very creative, because young people tend to have lateral minds, so it's useful to harness that resource, but equally it's very important to an organization to have stability and so that's where I think a mix can be very valuable if you have the old people.

I can think of a situation that we had, perhaps five or six years ago, when based on the idea that it was going to cost less money, we had a team of approximately 20 school leavers who were working in the warehouse here. We had enormous problems as

179

a result of that because the balance. At the moment the workforce in the warehouse are probably age range from, I would say, early twenties through to late fifties.

You know, they won't bring the system down or they can't do any major sort of damage, but there is this lack of confidence in using technology. This probably doesn't apply at the younger end, you see a lot of younger people are using computers at school, so I mean they are much more familiar with it. It's only with the older person, that I think is part of the problem and in other areas I think you've got this difficulty of people fitting in with the team that is there.

As a response to demographic pressures and because some of the above advantages of employing older people were coming to be recognized, some employers in our sample had begun to recruit a greater number of older workers (Taylor & Walker 1994). In our postal survey of employers 19 per cent were seeking to recruit more older workers although less than 10 per cent were encouraging later retirement or had phased retirement schemes in operation. In the words of one personnel manager:

Also we were very concerned about the demographic influences on costs of labour in the centre of Bristol, and one could see the school leaver population, the entrants, salaries being talked up time and time again, and we were getting the silly situation where school leavers were coming and saying "Oh well, I know someone down the road will pay 'x' and therefore I won't even consider your organization, although we recognize your training is the best, I am after the money." We were hearing this sort of nonsense.

Relations between the generations

We found some evidence of antagonism between younger and older workers. For example this might occur if a younger person perceived that an older person was marking time before retirement. This sometimes caused resentment among younger workers. In the words of one personnel manager:

If they've got the skills and they're pulling their weight I don't think there's any problem at all. It tends to be where there's someone that's just seeing out the last few years of their career, to get their full pension contribution and young people might feel that they're carrying them a little bit. I think that's where they tend to be a rub. So it's not so much to do with their age as opposed to how they're working is where there can be a bit of tension. But equally I would say that can apply to young people. If someone's not pulling their weight who is young there'll be resentment of them as well.

Another personnel manager felt that younger people probably considered older people to be too slow to take decisions and out of touch with the problems facing younger people. The policy of recruiting a greater number of older people by a major travel agency company had met with considerable resistance from staff in local branches. In fact, rather than try to educate staff, this pressure had led to the eventual withdrawal of the scheme. Concern over whether older people would fit in with younger people, rather than attempting to educate people regarding age issues, was a priority expressed by other respondents. A personnel manager in another private company stated that, if they were seeking to fill a post in an office staffed with younger people, they would ask older candidates if they would mind working with younger people. Similarly another employer was finding that, increasingly, their account executives were dealing with younger people: "if you have a 50 year old visiting a 25 year old, where one doesn't equate with the other, it can be counter productive for us". However, in other organizations we visited age issues formed part of equal opportunities training courses while another employer was attempting to educate line managers as to the value of recruiting older workers. In the words of the personnel manger:

We were, in fact, aware of the "demographic timebomb" two or three years before it became headline knowledge. On the basis that we were actually talking to schools and we were quite concerned to hear about the falling rolls. This company, in fact, its recruitment was almost entirely from school leavers, so it was quite clear that they just weren't going to be there. So we were actually moving towards a policy of employing older people way back in 1985/86. By persuasion, and it's taken several years, we've actually moved to that position I think we were lucky that we were in the business of taking on older employees in the Bristol area before everybody woke up to it. When they suddenly found there was a shortage of school leavers, everyone said "Oh yes we shall have to do something about it". But having identified it we actually were in there fairly early on. I think therefore we were early on actually able to persuade managers of the sense of this.

We did not specifically enquire about the attitudes of trade union officials and so obtained very few data on this issue. However, a personnel manager at a major manufacturer of processed foods reported that local union officials had tried to prevent the introduction of a policy on the grounds that it would reduce opportunities for younger people. In the words of the personnel manager:

> We did recognize within our factories division we had a shortage of engineers and that was primarily because we weren't getting the young people coming through. So we thought, well, why don't we actually look at taking some of our mature workforce, as we term them, and then giving them the opportunity to do an accelerated training so they can actually work in the skilled craft area. So it is a case where we're actually sort of positively looking at the group. Now, interestingly, when we actually put this forward at annual negotiations, we met a huge wall of resistance from the trade unions because they saw this as taking jobs away from young people and they thought that young people should be having priority in the company and we should be focusing our attention there.

Previous research on redundancy shows that trade union representatives are often keen to negotiate early retirement for older employees and, if possible, protect the jobs of younger ones (Westergaard et al. 1989). While some employers were sympathetic to the problem of discrimination against older workers there was a pervasive view that, when management considered it necessary, older people should make way for younger people. At a time of high unemployment it was not considered appropriate to be introducing policies to aid older workers. In contrast to the limited efforts to recruit and retain older people almost half of the employers we interviewed had an early retirement scheme in operation (Taylor & Walker 1994). For example one personnel manager felt that a period of phased retirement rather than an abrupt end to employment would benefit older workers. However, it was stated that, "with unemployment being so high and I think an awful lot of young people being out on the unemployment market, then I think it would be wrong to actually introduce that at the moment". Similarly another personnel manager felt that, as the age of 60 was the accepted age of retirement in the company, older people were more vulnerable to economic pressures rather than people who had twenty years of working life ahead of them. These findings contrast with the enthusiasm of older workers for greater choice in the age at which they retire and the manner in which they retired. Other employers used terms like "looking after the younger generation" and "the crises in the employment market for younger people at the moment" but such statements tended not to be made about older people. In fact the youth orientated culture of some companies contrasted (although the two cultures were likely to coexist) with the very common early retirement culture. However, this was a matter of some concern to other employers who had found that when a person could take retirement at 50 years of age (a common age in the organizations we surveyed), employees were beginning to wind down in their late forties.

Fears about mass unemployment had also led some employers to consider that older people "needed to make way for young people". Another employer also stated that "if you are looking to retraining people or perhaps moving them to another location, it's easier to do it with young people". As well as older people being considered more expendable it was felt by a few employers that younger people were more useful to the company as the recession ended. On the other hand our data analysis revealed little evidence of employers willing to question the morality of trading older for younger workers. In the words of three employers:

> I personally think in some cases yes because with the number of unemployed we have and also the number of university leavers, school leavers, who are struggling to get on that first career ladder, I think that there should come a time in people's minds when they think "well I have done my bit".

> We needed what we called a leaner and fitter sort of outfit and the thought was that the young people were going to be slightly more, I don't know if dynamic is the right word but let's say that.

At the present time it's interesting, because there are so many young people unemployed, and in that sense it may be that some of the younger people could benefit from the job more, but on the other hand people who have been with you for years, why should they be put on the scrap heap just because somebody else is after their job?

Conclusion

Our research has shown that older workers believe that employers value them for their experience while younger people are valued because of their skills with new technology, because they are considered to be more trainable, are thought likely to be with the company for longer and because they are cheaper to employ. Some older workers felt that employers' attitudes towards older workers were becoming more favourable. However, when seeking work older people in our sample had often found that employers discriminated in favour of younger people. This was particularly the case if a young person was doing the interviewing.

While there was support for the view that older people should make way for young people it was also felt that employment decisions should be based on who is the best person for the job. A large number of older people in our survey wanted to, or expected to, be allowed to work beyond the state pension ages. We have also found evidence that in some instances employers were encouraging women to work beyond the state retirement age although many women still expect to retire at 60. Of those people who think that they will be allowed to stay in work after the state pension age the majority state that this will be in the same job with the same hours. However, those people expecting to leave their present jobs at state pension age and expecting to seek some other kind of work are likely to favour part-time employment. Partial and flexible retirement programmes are favoured by many older workers. Some companies have instituted partial retirement programmes. On the negative side some workers feel trapped in jobs they do not enjoy but need to stay in for financial reasons.

We have shown that organizations, particularly private sector companies, were considerably more likely to be youth orientated than older worker orientated. While there was some sympathy for the position of older workers there was a tendency to put young people first in decisions about recruitment and retention. We have shown that, although many employers value the experience of older workers, when it comes to decisions about redundancy it is likely to be that group that is first in line.

Our research also indicates that life experience is considered useful by employers but it is the up-to-date skills of young people, particularly in the area of new technology, which are valued more highly by employers. This view is reflected in the attitudes of older workers who see themselves as less employable and as having few advantages over younger people.

In our surveys of older workers and employers we have uncovered evidence of hostility towards older people from managers. In our survey of employers we also found a limited amount of evidence of hostility not only from managers but also from younger staff, although other employers spoke of older people acting as mentor figures to younger colleagues. There was also a limited amount of evidence of age discrimination on the part of trade unions.

What do these findings tell us about workplace relations between the generations? Our results indicate that employers and older workers agree that, in general, employers favour young people although the older workers in our sample appear to have correctly perceived that some organizations are now more enthusiastic about employing older people than they have been previously. On the other hand, perhaps reflecting a growing awareness of equal opportunities issues, several older workers argued that both younger and older workers should be given an equal chance of finding employment, but few employers subscribed to this position. Most were youth orientated, as reflected in career paths that were available only to younger people.

A greater orientation towards the employment of younger people among employers was most obvious in attitudes towards retirement where the wishes of many older people were at odds with the practice of employers. While many older workers favoured the option of working longer and phasing their retirement, few employers had moved in the direction of offering phased or flexible retirement schemes. On the contrary youth unemployment seemed to have been a much more emotive issue for employers than unemployment among older people. Employers seemed to be much more prepared to sacrifice older workers in order to protect the jobs of young people. This is a perspective that is rooted in the past and is clearly at odds with the changing life-course.

Note

1. When this survey was conducted people aged over 59 years were denied training under Training for Work, the government's main training programme for the unemployed. Since 1993, partly in response to our research findings, the age limit has been increased to 63 years of age.

CHAPTER 9

Learning generations: age and education

Tom Schuller

Introduction

The mere presence in this volume of a chapter on learning is itself significant. Despite the verbal recognition given to life-long learning,
education is still very strongly associated with schooling in the public
mind and the policy mentality. In so far as that is now changing, the
shift is towards a concern with staying on rates of young people, the
enhanced role of further education colleges and the pressures on universities to take larger numbers of school and college leavers. Educational thinking is still very much geared to a preparatory conception
of education that links it closely to youth. If it is the case that adults
generally are still marginal shadowy figures in the classrooms, refec-
tories and planning bodies of the education system, a fortiori we can
suppose that older people are not regarded as mainstream clients by
educational policy-makers, providers or indeed by academic analysts.
Analysis of inequalities in access to British universities defined the
"relevant age group" for university entrance as the number of people
aged 18 in that year and went smoothly on: "This is not entirely satisfactory, mainly because it makes no allowance for the entry of mature
students. However, it is the most appropriate measure, and is used by
the DES" (Blackburn & Jarman 1993: 212). An excellent and substantial volume on social policies and older adults, co-edited since the
mid-1980s by the editor of this book (Phillipson & Walker 1986), contained nothing on education. It would be unfair to point to any such
omission as signalling indifference; I do not believe that every work of
social analysis should contain reference to every social group. But

there is real significance in the way that the notion of older adults as learners has so little purchase in the public mind. For learning implies, above all, development, of an intellectual, physical, technical, personal or spiritual kind; and the notion of development runs counter to many of the dominant images of older people where the only forms of change envisaged are negative ones.

How far older adults should be treated as a separate group, analytically or for the purposes of fashioning policy and provision, is an issue that does concern those who have taken an interest in this area. There is by now a reasonably well-established distinction drawn between educational gerontology, gerontological education and education for older adults (Peterson 1983, Glendenning 1990). But the question of what it is that marks out older learners – beyond chronological age – remains an important one. The substance of this chapter, which deals with both education and training, in one sense directly challenges the orthodox separation of older adults as "retired", by bringing vocational learning into the sphere of debate and refusing to accept that the education of older adults refers only to learning activities unrelated to the labour market. This is as much a challenge to educationalists who are still reluctant to look at learning as a whole, especially where it takes place in work or work-related settings, as it is to employers who dismiss the learning potential of their older members of staff. But in another sense it uses the example of older adults to suggest a reorientation of conventional approaches to education that is unrelated to employment, by stressing the investment function. (I discuss this below on page 193.) There is a two-way process of reconceptualization to be undertaken: to bring older people into the population of those recognized as learners and potential learners; and to expand the notion of what is regarded as learning and redefine its basis in social theory.

This chapter does not set out to cover in full that formidable stretch of ground. In a much more limited way it sets out to make use of the volume's focus on generational relations in the following way. Drawing on the results of the Carnegie Inquiry into the Third Age (1993) into the circumstances of Third Agers in the UK I shall report on the current position of older people in relation to learning opportunities, and how their access to learning compares with younger generations. I look at gender differences in access to education and training among older people and then widen the focus away from formal education and consider the question of how older men and women learn new roles in later life. Finally I explore some of the implications for intergenerational relations, and conclude by putting forward the notion of an intergenerational educational contract that would under-pin the promotion of an educational entitlement for adults.

The chapter is based largely on work done as part of the Carnegie Inquiry into the Third Age, which covered a wide range of policy areas affecting those aged 50 and over: employment, fiscal policy, health, volunteering, housing and so on. A summary report brought together the main conclusions and recommendations in a single vol-ume (Carnegie Inquiry into the Third Age 1993). The study on educa-tion, training and information was carried out at Edinburgh University's Centre for Continuing Education (Schuller & Bostyn 1992). Our study was broad brush and policy related. It brought together available information across a wide range, drawing on con-sultative inquiries with a number of different professional and consumer groups and concluding with a number of policy options. But this chapter also draws on other work on how older people learn new social roles. This study, which is qualitative and exploratory, involves interviews with a number of grandparents and seeks in par-ticular to explore differences – and similarities – between men and women in the way that they handle their new social position.

Learning in the third age: the economic and social context

Chronological age is relevant to learning ability and achievement. There is an association between age and, for example, the ability to memorize or the capacity to absorb information rapidly (Fry 1992). But the primary way in which age affects learning is in the prejudices it generates and the stereotypes it is used to support. These attitudes are displayed by policy-makers, employers, educators and by older people themselves (Midwinter 1992). The general conclusion to be drawn from the research literature and from the experience and reflections of those in the field is that we have barely begun to explore the complex learning potential of older people, and that this varies as much within this population as it does in any other broad age group. As Baltes et al. (1992: 157) observe, in a distillation of many years' research on ageing:

> . . . because of the underdeveloped state of a culture of old age, we know very little about the developmental potential of

189

older persons. As was true in earlier times for other age periods such as infancy and childhood, it will take an extended period of societal effort and much technological investment before the kind of differentiated culture of old age will have been reached that will uncover the latent potential of old age and empower older persons to choose among various opportunity structures.

Labour market positions are changing rapidly. The departure – forced or voluntary – of older men from the labour force has been analyzed at various levels (Walker et al. 1989, Young & Schuller 1991, Trinder et al. 1992). The scale of this trend means that pension and retirement ages no longer coincide and the duration of the working life becomes socially problematic in the sense that it is no longer based on widely accepted social norms. One consequence for intergenerational relations is a potential tension between older and younger workers over limited job opportunities. For a prime example one need look no further than the academic sphere, where younger scholars find their career paths apparently blocked by the preceding generation of tenured staff. I have nothing to say specifically on the issue of how far there is genuine competition for jobs, except to observe that the zero-sum approach – that the more jobs are taken away from one generation the more employment there will be for another – is sterile and limited in the extreme. But there are concrete and significant, if often unappreciated, consequences for the attitudes and policies adopted towards older people when it comes to workplace learning opportunities. On the part of both individual and employer it makes sense to invest in training only if there is a fair chance of a return to the investment. Expectations that older workers should make way for younger ones will therefore militate against the provision of training for them; conversely, for an employer to provide training for older employees is a statement of a kind about intention to continue their employment, and possibly also to provide career prospects for them. In other words, for older people to have access to training implies not only that their work is valued but also that they have a future in the occupation.

This becomes particularly important when we look at the changing structure of employment. The sectoral shifts that have been occurring since the early 1970s are familiar. Most of these, notably the shift away from manufacturing and engineering, have affected older, and often unskilled, males most severely. This is thoroughly documented in the work done for the Carnegie Inquiry by the Institute for Employment Research (IER). Their projections show a decline in the number of males over 55 in employment of some 241,000 between 1990 and 2000, and an increase in female employment of some 149,000 (Lindley et al. 1991 Table 2.1). As a proportion of the older workforce, women will rise, though not greatly, from 34 per cent in 1971 to 39 per cent in 2000. This is part of a wider and deeper trend; International Labour Organization (ILO) figures show activity rates for women aged 45–54 in the most developed regions rose from 43 per cent in 1950 to 63 per cent in 1980, and are predicted to reach 66 per cent by 2000 (Standing 1986). Such growth as will occur in the employment of older workers is likely to be largely concentrated in part-time jobs, characteristically but not exclusively held by females, and usually offering little in the way of training.

I turn now from the labour market to an extremely summary presentation of the principal social changes that affect the position of older people as learners in the context of intergenerational analysis. First is the tighter focus on job-related training as the main recipient of government expenditure on learning. This means that some of the main types of educational provision that appeal to older people are under threat, despite having been an integral part of welfare provision over a number of decades. Local authority classes, which are the largest organized form of adult education and especially important for older people, are particularly vulnerable – a threat which is made even more menacing by the possible intention to levy VAT on adult education provision that is deemed to be "recreational". Secondly, the growth of the segment of the population designated as the "very old" has begun to draw attention to the issue of caring and what the respective contributions of professionals and other, unpaid, workers should be. Implicated here are a whole cluster of issues involving individuals of different ages, as potential carers and as potential dependants. These affect intergenerational relations both at the macro-level, in the implications for public expenditure, and at the micro-level in the impact on personal and familial circumstances. In other words all (or most) of us are affected by tax and benefit transfers across generations, and many of us may be personally affected by the services provided as part of public policy and by the social obligations and responsibilities generated as a result. Pessimistic scenarios have been painted of a far greater burden falling on unsupported relatives.

Surprisingly little attention has been paid to preventive policies, especially those not specifically designated as relating to physical health.

Thirdly, the work carried out by older people as volunteers often involves significant, but equally often unrecognized, levels of skill – including the acquisition of new skills (Davis Smith 1992). Economic assessments of the value of this work vary greatly depending on the methodology employed, but it can plausibly be estimated as running into billions of pounds annually. Imprecise though the quantifications may be, to the value of the services provided there should be added the accumulation and conservation of human capital through volunteering: people carry on using skills that would otherwise have been lost, and develop new ones that have application beyond the immediate context of the volunteer work.

All of these signal the need for what we have called a "social economy of the Third Age" (Schuller & Bostyn 1992: 86), which would recognize the actual and potential contributions made by older people, and the need for corresponding investment in learning opportunities. This would mark a radical shift in public conceptions of adult education. As Moody (1993: 224) observes, policy on older adult education has taken a wrong strategic turn:

> The strategic error has both an economic and a social component. In terms of economic policy, older-adult education has favored consumption rather than production. . . . It is constructed as a form of leisure-time activity, not human-capital investment. In terms of social policy, older-adult education has developed almost entirely separately from the "aging enterprise" activities of human services, including health care, social welfare and the formal aging network. . . . This strategic orientation towards individual learning outside of social structure has had devastating results for older-adult education, depriving it of any wider legitimation. The concept of productive aging could offer a wider alternative.

Despite holding reservations about the concept of productive ageing (reservations that are given powerful articulation by Holstein 1993) I concur with Moody in the need for a strategic shift in the approach to learning by older adults, a shift that gives proper place to their actual and potential contributions, measured not only in economic terms but also in the overall impact on society of the presence of people with experience and the opportunity to have that experience valued.

The notion of strategy has temporal implications that may appear to conflict with the notion of investment as the key to policy for older adults. Human capital theory, which in its less crude forms has much to offer analysts of educational policy, has in the past been used to favour bringing investment as far forward as possible in the life-course, in order for the returns to be payable over as long a period as possible. On this line of reasoning, adults, and especially older adults, have a far lesser claim on educational resources than young people. There are at least three counter-arguments to this. First, while there will always be competition for resources, investment in older adults need not be at the expense of youth. Secondly, investment in learning opportunities, broadly conceived, for older adults is at least likely to bring about a saving in other forms of expenditure. To put it at its crudest: if participation in a class postpones for even one week the entry of an individual into the state of dependency that requires residential care it will have paid for itself something like ten times over. Thirdly, the so-called payback periods for training are shortening, as organizational and technological change occurs. Ironically, given the supposed antipathy between older people and change, this substantially improves the case for investment, since older people will not have to work, or live, for as long as previously (implicitly) calculated to "justify" the investment.

I have put these arguments baldly simply in order to provide a framework of some kind for judging the adequacy of current provision. In the Carnegie study we propose other dimensions for measuring that elusive notion, including international comparisons, rising expectations, social distribution and the quality of provision (Schuller & Bostyn 1992: 9–10). I turn now to the evidence from the study itself on the actual distribution of formal learning opportunities.

Current participation

Our brief for the Carnegie Inquiry was a broad one: to give an account of the existing patterns of education, training and information; to identify the main issues and concerns in these areas; and to provide policy options. We began by analyzing the position in respect of formal education – organized classes – and worked our way outwards, through training and into the very diffuse and disparate field of information and informal learning. The work covered people still in paid employment and with possibly another two decades of such work, and people who had long since finished employment or had never been employed. In other words it covered several generations, as defined both by chronological age and by reference to social or labour market position.

Both conceptualizing and measuring intergenerational inequality is a philosophical and methodological minefield. Temkin (1992), pursuing a line of argument raised by McKerlie, points to three primary and significantly different forms of egalitarianism. The *complete lives* egalitarian looks at the distribution of opportunities or expenditure over the entire life-times of the individuals to be compared. The *simultaneous segments* egalitarian chooses historical or chronological periods as the basic unit, contrasting people's experience within that unit regardless of their age or stage. Thus the access of different age groups to health care, or to education, is compared for a given year or number of years, regardless of the fact that the propensity to make use of these services may vary as a function of age. The *corresponding stage* egalitarian, by contrast, chooses to compare people who are at the same stage or age, though this may be located at different historical times – in other words, the comparison is between 30–40 year old cohorts, or adolescents, or maturescents, at different historical periods. The outcomes of any intergenerational analysis can, obviously, vary greatly according to which of these approaches is deployed.

Table 9.1 gives details of the current distribution of qualifications across age groups. It shows the dramatic imbalance in the levels of formal qualification, especially in the proportions of the different age groups who have no formal qualification at all. Nearly two-thirds of those aged 60–69 have no qualifications at all, compared with less than one-fifth of those aged 20–29. It should be remembered that this shows not only that older people almost all left school at the minimum age, but also that in the intervening four or five decades they have been unable to acquire any formal certification of their skills or expertise.

Different generations have different levels of access to education and training throughout their lives. Table 9.2 is based on Labour Force Survey data and gives details of access to training by age group. From one angle it shows clearly that initial inequalities are more likely to increase over time. In particular, those without skills – and therefore

194

Table 9.1 Highest qualification by age group (%).

	20–29	30–39	40–49	50–59	60–69	Difference old–young
Degree or equivalent	8	11	8	5	5	–3
Higher education below degree level	9	13	11	9	6	–3
GCE A level or equivalent	15	11	7	4	2	–13
GCE O level or equivalent/ CSE Grade 1	34	23	16	10	6	–28
CSE other grades/ commercial qualifications/ apprenticeship	15	9	11	11	12	–3
Foreign or other qualifications	2	3	4	4	3	1
No qualifications	18	30	44	57	65	47

Source: Office of Population Censuses and Surveys 1990: Table 7.5

most vulnerable to economic change – are least likely to have opportunities to train or retrain, except if they become unemployed. (Older
workers, however, do not benefit to the same extent from training
schemes for the unemployed: they participate at lower rates, and the
outcome for them is more likely to be a return to unemployment, even
if they do not actually claim unemployment benefit.) However, Table
9.3. shows how, in the context of Temkin's typology, we have different
tendencies at work. For the corresponding segment egalitarian the
position is improving, as a higher proportion of older people gain
access to training of some kind. 55 year olds in 1990 had a higher
probability of receiving training than 55 year olds in 1984. For the
simultaneous segment egalitarian, by contrast, the inequalities are
actually increasing over time, as younger cohorts gain more in the
general growth in training opportunities. Thus the proportion of
those in the Second Age (aged between 25 and 49) who had received
training in the previous four weeks rose by nearly seven percentage
points, from 8.6 per cent to 15.3 per cent in the period concerned,
while the rise in the proportion of 55–59 year olds was of 4.2 percentage points only.

One of the awkward features, but at the same time one of the major
strengths, of the Carnegie study on learning is its inclusion of both
education and training. Obviously people are not only employees but

Table 9.2   Received job training in previous four weeks (%).

	First age (under 25)		Second age (25–49)		Third age (50–59/64)	
	M	F	M	F	M	F
Employed only						
Degree equivalent	36	38	25	32	15	28
A level	28	26	12	17	6	10
O level	28	21	13	14	8	10
No qualifications	11	8	5	5	3	3
All respondents	25	22	13	15	7	8
Manual	21	17	7	6	3	2
Non-manual	31	25	20	19	10	12
Leads to qualification?	70	68	33	35	10	19
Length six months+	71	67	28	20	9	31

Source: Department of Employment 1992

Table 9.3   Received job training in last four weeks (% of all dependent employees).

	1984			1986			1988			1990		
	Total	M	F	Total	M	F	Total	M	F	Total	M	F
All ages	9.1	9.6	8.4	10.7	11.4	9.9	13.2	13.3	13.0	15.3	15.2	15.5
First Age	16.0	18.5	13.2	18.2	20.7	15.5	20.1	22.0	18.1	22.0	23.7	20.2
Second Age	8.6	9.1	7.9	10.1	10.9	9.2	13.0	13.2	12.8	15.3	15.0	15.6
Pre-retirement	3.1	3.0	3.4	4.0	3.8	4.2	5.5	5.0	6.3	7.7	7.3	8.3
Post-retirement	2.2	–	2.2	2.5	–	2.5	1.5	–	1.5	–	–	–
50-54	4.1	4.2	4.0	5.2	5.1	5.3	6.6	6.2	7.0	9.6	9.4	9.8
55-9	2.4	2.2	2.7	3.2	3.4	3.0	5.2	5.0	5.4	6.6	6.8	6.4
60-64	2.0	2.0	–	2.3	2.3	–	2.7	2.7	–	4.0	4.0	–
All under 3A	10.6	11.6	9.5	12.4	13.5	11.0	14.9	15.5	14.3	17.0	17.1	16.8

Source: Labour Force Survey 1990

also citizens, and learn for many different reasons of which occupational ones are only one set. The results quoted above, showing the generally very low levels of training provided for older workers, should not be interpreted only in relation to older people as workers. People bring to their life after work attitudes and habits from the workplace; to be specific, people who are learning at work are more likely to carry on learning after work, whether this is on a daily basis or in a life-cycle context. Those who cross the threshold of the Third

Age without what might be called the learning habit are very much less likely to acquire it subsequently. Training practices therefore affect very much more than the immediate economic performance of the individual concerned. Without access to learning on the job, learning off, and after, the job becomes more difficult. The contrast with succeeding generations, where learning is becoming part of the job (and where job change and the learning that goes with it is more common), is striking.

There is, however, another respect in which the inequalities of previous ages are to some extent redressed later on in life. In both education and training, older women appear to enjoy significantly greater access to learning than their male counterparts. This phenomenon is quite well known in adult education, but the figures on training are much more surprising. Participation by older women in adult education is stronger well before they begin to outnumber men significantly in the population as a whole, at about 70. Age data were available from England for enrolments in many though not all of the classes run in further education colleges. Here there has been a strong growth in enrolments by people aged 50 and over. Most of these are in non-vocational classes, and women outnumber men by something like two to one.

The data on training (Table 9.2) show that a highly qualified older woman has a better chance of receiving training than even a similarly qualified younger man, and a very much better chance than any men of her own age. Thus 28 per cent of older women with a degree or equivalent qualification had received some form of job training in the previous four weeks, compared with 15 per cent of older men and 25 per cent of younger men. Of course the numbers of highly qualified older women in the workforce are quite small, but the figures are significant and the pattern applies across different levels of qualification, except for the wholly unqualified, where men and women are equally badly off, with only 3 per cent getting training of any kind in a given year.

One explanation suggested for this partial rebalancing of unequal gender access to training has been that it is accounted for by older women entering jobs that require some minimal technical training, such as counter clerks in financial institutions. This interpretation is belied by the last line of Table 9.2, which shows that of those who participated in training a far higher proportion of women than men were involved over a substantial period, defined as six months or more.

197

This does not necessarily mean that the training was full-time during the period concerned, but it does exclude the half-day induction to a computer as an explanation, and makes more detailed investigation of the types of training received an issue of interest and significance. I shall return to the gender issue, from a rather different angle, later in the chapter.

Future demand and intergenerational influences

In the Carnegie report we suggest that there will be a steep increase in the demand for learning on the part of older people, for a number of reasons. The rise in overall educational levels in the population as a whole is certain to generate new demands for continuing education, and to modify public and personal perceptions of learning potential. As average educational levels (measured, crudely, by length of schooling and possession of formal qualifications) rise, so people moving into later life will challenge the barriers that excluded earlier generations from many forms of learning, while later generations, with more schooling behind them, are still better equipped to take advantage of learning opportunities. (The pattern can be clearly observed even in a country like Sweden, with a longstanding public commitment to social equality and impressive record on adult education: see Rubenson 1989.) Other factors include changes in the social and economic climate that are gradually, if belatedly, bringing about an acknowledgement of education as a life-long process. Government and industry are setting targets that should push and pull more people into continuing education and remove at least some of the institutional and attitudinal barriers preventing adults from participating in learning.

These targets will not be easy to achieve. One line of argument is to suggest that resources and efforts should be concentrated on the young. Unsurprisingly I would reject this, and not only on grounds of equity. Financial incentives (and disincentives), labour market prospects and the attractiveness of the educational experience are the major immediate factors that will affect the participation rates of younger students. But in the medium term we are talking about a change in culture. Whilst older people may not have a direct and explicit influence on younger people's decisions, the implicit example of older generations returning to learn is potentially powerful, and will make it easier for younger generations to find a way back into learning.

I want to add one point of a more speculative nature that may nevertheless prove influential on patterns of demand. It is well established that the initial educational achievements of young people are strongly influenced by the educational levels of their parents, whether this is in staying on at school beyond the minimum school leaving age or in securing access to higher education. It seems at least plausible that a reverse process may also be beginning to be at work, namely that as older people see their children and even grandchildren benefiting from education they may in turn be encouraged to take part themselves. In other words, there may be a process of filial as well as parental influence at work that will reinforce those other factors to which we have pointed. At present there is only the occasional photograph of parents and children brandishing certificates received at the same degree ceremony; the wider picture needs to be sketched in. Research into the dynamics of intergenerational relations would do well to hypothesize reverse or mutual influences of this kind (Schuller 1993).

Learning new roles: grandfathering and grandmothering
It is only since the mid-1980s that the intersection of age and gender is beginning to assume any significance in social science (Phillipson & Walker 1986, Arber & Ginn 1991). Research at the Centre for Continuing Education has explored the ways in which men and women conceive of and adapt to the role of grandparent, based on interviews with about thirty grandparents in the Edinburgh area (Bamford 1993, 1994). One objective was to set formal learning, of the type referred to earlier in this chapter, alongside the kind of informal learning that entry into a new role mainly involves. This is a small scale study in a field with major sociological and psychological implications that seem hardly to have been addressed, but a number of issues can be provisionally identified as significant.

Changes in demographic and family structures are leading to a far more complex system of intergenerational relations. Increased longevity means increased numbers of grandparents and great-grandparents, while higher divorce rates mean that the relations are more seldom of a simple linear vertical kind. For many older people, becoming a grandparent is an event of major significance, especially if they have finished paid employment, but the emotional and social

199

parameters of grandparenting have not been much examined (Bengston & Robertson 1985). Being a grandparent can involve a joyous relationship between a first and a third generation; but it also has many other implications, especially for the relationship between grandparent and parent.

For all children, and especially for all adults, much of the learning that takes place is informal (Tough 1983). Educational institutions play a part in helping people to acquire knowledge, skills and values, but are only one of a number of influences on development. Those who become grandparents usually learn the role intuitively. Most of our interviewees were born in the 1920s and 1930s, and learned their parenting role also intuitively, well before sex education was established in schools and also before much learning was passed down within families. Nevertheless the following case illustrates how powerful the example of a grandparent can be:

> Jean did not feel loved or understood in her immediate family. Her happy childhood memories were of times spent with her grandmother, not her mother, and she still can't remember her grandmother without tears. I asked her whether she had learned anything from her, and she replied, "Just trying to be kind to people. She was very kind." Her grandmother had provided a refuge for Jean, a place where she felt special: "Every time I fell out with my mother I would be up to my grandmother to get some sympathy there. She never criticized my mother. She was very good about that, but she always thought that I was in the right."

Jean, like several of the women we interviewed, had suffered because her mother had favoured the boys in the family. Jean, learning from the negative in the way her mother treated her, and the positive from her grandmother's interest and concern, has always tried to encourage her daughters to be assertive, and to maintain a warm and close relationship with them. Now she is a grandmother she is ready to be the "bolthole" that she needed as a child, but is thankful that her grandchildren are happy in their day-to-day lives, and come to visit her not for solace but for fun (Bamford 1994, Ch. 1).

Other interviewees referred to ways in which they had learned how to be a grandparent from the way a particular grandparent had been with them, for example in helping them through unhappy childhoods. Yet the gap between being a small grandchild and becoming a grandparent is obviously many times greater than that between being a child and a parent. Role models, good or bad, are less immediately available. Alexander, one of the men in our study, recalled a grandfather who was a minister and a widower:

He used to have his porridge in the morning, he had no electricity originally, all paraffin lamps, so one learnt how to deal with paraffin lamps. He had log fires, he used to get sleepers from the railway and cut them up himself. . . . Right, one went down and helped with these things so one learned a great deal from one's grandparents, and one learned that things don't come just like that, you've got to go and do things yourself, you have to apply yourself and work. (Bamford 1994, Ch. 1)

Alexander, it was clear, had learned much from his ancestor, and some of the clarity of rules had stayed with him; but how far the man acted as an example of a grandfather to him is less certain. The men in the study welcomed the erosion of gender divisions and weakening of gender stereotypes. "None of them spoke out for the patriarchal father and grandfather of old – he was recalled as a forbidding, and often unhappy, figure" (Bamford 1994, Ch. 6).

The socialization process by which people learn to become grandparents is fragmentarily understood. It may at times involve significant resocialization, as grandparents come to accept that it is their children who are the parents now, and who are primarily responsible for the normative education of the latest generation.

They may have disapproved of their child's choice of spouse, or of their daughters becoming single parents, or, as we shall see, of their child-rearing styles, but they found ways to contain any of their disagreements, and several talked of how they had learned from the ways their children and grandchildren were living their lives. Some people coped by recognizing that the modern world cannot be lived in in outdated ways. Irene expressed this well:

I think very often, they're living in different times. The whole world has changed so fast, that for our generation it's quite hard to absorb it. I don't think you can criticise too much, or interfere, without being out there with the problem. . . . I would hate to be bringing up teenagers in this day and age. (Bamford 1994, Ch. 1)

201

In some instances, this process of resocialization may involve quite profound reconsideration of the older person's own behaviour as parent, in respect both of the past and the present.

In practice, James, like Nicholas, had worked long hours when his children were growing up, and he had not given the time to his children that he sees his son, and his son's friends, giving now. Unlike Nicholas, who feels no regret at his absences from the home, James does wish that he had been more like his son:

> . . . if I look at my son, the time and care that he devotes to his son it is considerably greater than I, and I think most fathers of my generation did manage to have. The role of husbands and fathers has changed, and they now play a greater, more equal part in day-to-day domestic and family activities. It's not that someone like my son has any more time from his work than I had for looking after children and dealing with domestic chores, rather it's because changed attitudes have made such partnership more customary than in the past. (Bamford 1994: 60–61)

Thus grandparents may learn about parenting from their own children, as well as teaching them explicitly or implicitly.

For this generation in particular, such learning may involve considerable changes in behaviour, and this may be especially true of grandfathers. Men who played the traditional role of fathers find themselves in a new role that involves them affectively in ways that were unfamiliar to them as fathers.

> I used to wonder about old men who went all ga ga about their grandchildren. When I became a grandfather, I saw what it was. Marvellous. It's a privilege to be a grandparent. There's no question about it. It's a privilege. It gave me back something I'd missed. I'd missed all these formative years with my own children. (Bamford 1994: 24)

As parents they had a clear if complex normative responsibility, to which the affective side may often have been sacrificed; as grandparents this normative role is replaced by a less clear one of affective availability.

Some of this verges on psychological speculation, but there are substantial educational and sociological implications. One major one, alluded to several times in the passages quoted above, is the way grandparenting is part of a more general shift in gender relations in later life. Gutmann (1987) has applied psychological tests to populations in a number of different cultures that suggest that the values and attitudes exhibited by men and women come closer together in later life, with men becoming more affective and women more "agentic". This opens up many potentially fruitful avenues for exploration, especially in the relationship between paid and unpaid work and the values assigned to different forms of activity as people move into later stages of the life-course. Grandparenting may be one such activity alongside full- or part-time employment, voluntary work and hobbies or recreation. What sort of changes occur in the ways in which men and women combine these different activities, and how are they enabled to carry them out to the full? Each involves a set of skills, some of which may already have been learnt, but some of which are there to be acquired, formally or informally. Included in this already formidable list are the challenges posed by changing personal relationships among older people, as well as between them and those of other generations.

Conclusion: towards an intergenerational educational contract

The Carnegie study attempts to bring together formal and informal learning into a common framework. Its point of departure is that older people need access to learning opportunities just as much as any other group in order to change and develop successfully. Intergenerational analysis has two key functions. The first is to reveal differences in the ways in which different generations have effective access to learning opportunities, formal or informal, and to set this in a historical context that takes account of accumulated inequalities. The second is to clarify the way in which successive generations are or might be involved in learning from and with each other, either as part of a set of family relationships or simply as participants and collaborators. The notion of "generation" can be used to denote a relationship between different age groups, or to identify one such group or to refer to a particular span of time. All these are intrinsically diffuse and changing, which makes the task difficult but intriguing.

The status of an intergenerational contract is a complex matter that can be approached from many different angles. What I am proposing here is something quite simple in outline. One generation contributes to the economic development of a country, and this is taken as justifying its right to a decent standard of living in old age. Whether or not the contract is honoured, and the criteria to be used in assessing the equity of the contract do not concern us here. But just as the generation contributes to the formation of physical capital, so it contributes to the formation of human capital, through the financing of formal education systems and through the socialization and informal education of the young. An intergenerational educational contract would recognize the rights of older people to the fruits of such developments, not in the form of financial maintenance but through access to learning opportunities. In this line of thinking, a "pension" would comprise not just a regular weekly payment, but an entitlement to avail oneself of the chance of personal development.

This basic proposition is buttressed by two considerations, both mooted earlier in the chapter. First is the argument that the student population as a whole gains from participation by older people – "student" here being used in the broad sense to include informal learners as well as those enrolled in formal classes. Secondly, the entitlement should not be seen merely as a form of licensed expenditure, to be registered on the debit side of any account. The spending power of pensioners is an important component of the economy as a whole. Similarly, expenditure on the development of older people brings its own returns, some but not all of which are translatable into economic terms. Thus many of those past state pension age already continue in some kind of paid employment, and this proportion is likely to rise in the future. Voluntary activity, including caring for others, is a major unrecorded contribution to the prosperity of the country that would be enhanced by better educational provision. Furthermore – and here we enter the realm of the unquantifiable – older people play an important role as what Laslett (1989) has called "cultural trustees", including civic and political life. All these components of the social economy of the Third Age make the contract not a one-way but a two-way transaction. For each "pair" of generations, the older is giving in the present, as well as receiving in return for its past efforts. The validity of the contract does not depend on the balance being neutral at any given time – in other words, that older people should in some sense be paying back as much as they get in educational terms – but it signals that there is some actual reciprocity at work.

I conclude with a policy recommendation to give substance to the notion of the intergenerational educational contract. In the Education Act 1944 there was a proposal to make day release compulsory for those who left school at the minimum age. This was never implemented. The generation that failed to benefit from this measure is now entering the Third Age. There would therefore be a particular historical resonance to a measure that gave older people, especially those who had had least initial education, some kind of specific educational entitlement. Day release as such would not be an appropriate form for such an entitlement since the temporal rhythms of older people are not the same as young people on a weekly wage. But a measure that enabled, say, everyone as they reached the age of 50 to support for time off work to learn something, and for those not in paid employment to benefit similarly, would be a solid indication of a social valuing of the potential of older people. This is not fanciful; in the Carnegie report we cite the example of an American employer that does just that (including, for good measure, the spouse in the entitlement). And if it acted as a stalking horse for the introduction of a more general entitlement, this would be a perfect vindication for the idea of a contract that would be of mutual benefit to the participating generations.

CHAPTER 10

Intergenerational conflict and the welfare state: American and British perspectives

Chris Phillipson

Introduction

In 1949 the Royal Commission on Population delivered its report on the long-term future of the population of Great Britain. The background to the work of the Commission was the concern, expressed throughout the 1930s and 1940s, about the possible dangers arising from the ageing of the population. In this debate older people were depicted as a burden on society; a group with the potential for reducing the living standards of the nation and increasing the financial pressures on future generations of workers. The Royal Commission expressed particular anxiety about the conflict of interest between workers and pensioners. The basis for this concern was expressed in the Commission's view that:

> ... if all the old sit back on their first pensionable birthday and draw a pension with which they compete for consumer goods made by a decreasing section of the population, the standard of life of both generations will inevitably be endangered. (Royal Commission on Population 1949)

The concept of generations competing over scarce resources was underplayed during the 1950s and 1960s in Britain which, in common with many other industrial societies, fashioned new approaches to the provision of welfare (Lowe 1993). However, by the 1970s and 1980s, the notion of generational conflict was back on the political agenda and had become a major topic of debate within and beyond the gerontological community (Easterlin 1978, Clark & Spengler 1980, Foote 1982, Longman 1987, Johnson et al. 1989, Phillipson 1990, Walker 1990a, Hobman 1993).

The terms of this more recent debate have not been substantially different from that initiated by the Royal Commission in the late 1940s. For example, in his influential article "Children and the elderly in the US", the demographer Samuel Preston (1984) raised the possibility of direct competition between young and old over the distribution of economic resources. From a social as well as economic perspective, Preston argued that it was difficult to justify curtailing expenditure on children. Echoing the views of the Royal Commission, Preston argued: "Whereas expenditure on the elderly can be thought of mainly as consumption, expenditure on the young is a combination of consumption and investment". And he went to highlight the possibility of increasing polarization in the provision of social policy, concluding:

> If we care about our collective future rather than simply about our future as individuals we are faced with the question of how best to safeguard the human and material resources represented by children. These resources have not been carefully guarded in the past two decades. (Preston 1984: 49)

The concern of this chapter is not to review the empirical basis for arguments about "generational equity" (these are covered in Chs 1 and 3), and numerous articles are available reviewing different perspectives on the debate.[1] Instead the purpose of this chapter is, first, to examine the different ways in which the question of generational equity may be approached; secondly, to assess the meaning of key concepts used in the discussion; thirdly, to examine some of the issues raised by the debate for the future organization of the welfare state.[2]

Interpreting the debate on population ageing

How, first of all, do we make sense of the anxieties about population ageing and the question of equity between generations? Clearly, the approach taken by researchers will reflect the concerns and perspectives of their individual disciplines. In respect of the social sciences, Johnson & Falkingham (1992) have usefully detailed three main approaches. From an economic perspective, the concern has been with problems that may arise from the transfer of resources between generations. In a context of declining worker–pensioner ratios, the questions raised by researchers have focused upon the fairness of such transfers and the influence they may have on incentives to work or save. The policy implications have been identified in terms of limiting tax burdens, curbing expenditure on social programmes, and increasing the supply of labour. According to Johnson & Falkingham (1992: 178): "In most of the economic analysis of population ageing, the welfare of older people in the future appears (if at all) as very definitely subservient to the goal of effective macroeconomic management".

Secondly, in the case of social policy, the dominant concerns have historically been with the welfare of older people and the development of policies to improve relative living standards. Social policy analysts have also provided a critique of the "public-burden concept of welfare", claiming that the concern about population ageing has been influenced by ideologically driven policies aimed at reducing the state's role in welfare (Binney & Estes 1988, Walker 1990a, Minkler & Robertson 1991). The policy implications of this approach have been to develop a counter-ideology based on the concept of interdependence between generations (Kingson et al. 1986) as well as proposing action to improve the living standards of the present generation of older people (Bornat et al. 1985, Estes 1992, Walker 1990a).

Thirdly, from a sociological perspective there has been a broader assessment of the transformation in social relationships reflected in an ageing society. Featherstone & Hepworth (1988) have described these changes as part of the modernization of ageing, with factors such as the growth in early retirement, the emergence of distinctive life-styles among older people, and the renegotiation of relationships between old and young within the sphere of the family. From a policy perspective, these changes are seen to raise fundamental questions about the status of older people and their integration in society. Older people, it is argued, have gained free time and longevity but lead marginal and often trivialized lives (Moody 1988, Cole 1992). To challenge this crisis of old age, it is argued that we must reassess both the meanings attached to later life (through, for example, an attack on age discrimination) and increase the power and status of the old within economic, social and cultural institutions (Laczko & Phillipson 1991, Young & Schuller 1991).

Finally, we should note also the work of historians such as Cole (1992) and Achenbaum (1974, 1978), who have helped provide a broader perspective on interpretations of demographic change. Cole points out that the late twentieth century is not the first era to turn its disappointments and anxieties into anger against old age. His research suggests that amidst the late-nineteenth-century crisis of Victorian morality and the decline of classical liberalism, old age in the USA came to be viewed as an intractable barrier to the limitless accumulation of health and wealth. The theme of the "obsolescence of old age", to use Achenbaum's (1974) phrase, became widespread and fed into a devaluation of the aged in comparison to the young. One hundred years later, society was again haunted by the "specter of an ageing society". Cole argues that:

In the late twentieth century, old age has again emerged as a lightning rod for the storms of liberal capitalism and of middle-class identity. This time, it is the middle-aged baby boomers who are most susceptible to neo-conservative Cassandras who forecast intergenerational Armageddon and the bankruptcy of the federal government. Fears about declining fertility and the burden of an ageing population merge with the fiscal and ideological crises of the welfare state. Personal anxieties about growing old are conflated with pessimism about the future. Critics and commentators represent the aging of our social institutions with metaphors of decline, exhaustion, and collapse. (Cole 1992, 235)

These different interpretations of ageing have areas both of complementarity as well as conflict. Taking the former, economists have provided important contributions to evaluating issues relating to dependency ratios, pension provision, and policies for work and retirement (Schulz 1988). The perspective of social policy is especially important both in highlighting the heterogeneity of the old in terms of income and wealth (Phillipson 1993), as well as identifying future options for the development of the welfare state (Hills 1993). The contribution from sociology has helped to highlight the nature of ageing as a reflexive process; that is, its capacity to change social institutions as well as be changed by them. Finally, historians have pointed to the dualism in social images of old age: ageing simultaneously, or at different times, represented as a period of social decay or social progress.

At the same time, the areas of conflict between particular disciplines need to be clarified, if not resolved, if the debate on generational equity is to progress. The main focus of this chapter is to critically examine the concept of generations and the related issue of generational equity. The discussion will be offered from the perspective of a sociologist using the literature on the nature of generations and the possibilities it offers for re-evaluating the significance of population change.

Generational change and conflict

A crucial element in the debate about population ageing has been the use of the concept of generations as a way of explaining both current and potential problems facing the welfare state. Older people have been depicted as a "selfish welfare generation" (Thomson 1989) or "greedy geezers" (*New Republic* 28 March 1988), in the more direct language of North Americans, soaking the young whilst running up huge public expenditure deficits. In the area of health care, the bio-medical ethicist Callahan (1987) started an intense debate in the USA, following the publication of his book *Setting limits: medical goals in an ageing society*. His book identified three aspirations for an ageing society: first, to stop pursuing medical goals that combine the features of high costs, marginal gains, and benefits (in the main) for the old; secondly, that the old shift their priorities from their own welfare to that of younger generations; and thirdly, that older people should accept death as a condition of life, at least for the sake of others. Callahan's intervention attracted considerable critical debate and dissension (see, especially, Homer & Holstein 1990, Moody 1992) but it fuelled an already highly charged debate concerning the divergent interests and attainments of young and old.

Underpinning the debate is a further concern that older people have begun to mobilize their electoral resources to press the case for additional benefits. Whilst difficult to argue in the case of Britain (see below), this has been a popular theme in the USA, where Marmor et al. (1990) note that, if the tales of journalists are to be believed, congressional representatives live in fear of arousing the displeasure of the American Association of Retired Persons (AARP).

All of this literature and research begs some crucial questions about the issue of generations as a sociological as opposed to economic concept. Economists are right, within their own terms, to point to the problems associated with resource transfers across generations.

210

Clearly, important issues need to be faced regarding how resources are allocated and the likely impact on different social groups. But the question that must also be pursued is whether the framing of these issues in generational terms clarifies or obscures the way in which relations between generations might develop. From a sociological perspective, the questions that must be asked include: how reliable is the idea of generations as a predictor of social and political action? Do people behave as if members of distinctive generations? And if they do, does this point to conflict or co-operation in the years ahead?

The problem of generations

At the heart of our problem is that an economic generation and a sociological generation are two distinct entities. With the former, issues are presented in terms of discrete groups competing – selfishly or otherwise – for a fair share of resources. At its most extreme, this model suggests that generations behave as if on a collision course, with the block votes of the old threatening to cut off services needed by the young (Longman 1987), and the young reconsidering the basis of the welfare contract and supporting threats to dismantle the welfare state (Thomson 1989). This last point has been expressed by Thomson in the following way:

> ... the very nature of aged populations is changing, in ways not comprehended in our present debates, and along with this come shifts in relations between generations. Members of the welfare generation are now arriving at old age with assets, expectations and histories of benefits quite unlike those of their predecessors, and it remains to be seen whether the young who are expected to make growing transfers to them will feel bound to do so. At the end of the twentieth century the implicit welfare contract that binds members of successor generations is up for renegotiation – and the aged stand right at the centre of this with a great deal to lose. (Thomson 1989: 35)

Of course, we might note the point made by Riley et al. (1972) that diverse tendencies do not necessarily become manifest in antagonism nor erupt into organized conflict. They comment: "The mere fact of inequality among age strata (as is true of other types of stratification also) is not a sufficient condition for age cleavage" (Riley et al. 1972: 443). In reality, the sociological generation will almost certainly behave in a more complex way than suggested by the worker versus pensioner perspective.

What do the sociologists mean when they use the term generations? Abrams (1982), in his classic essay "Identity and the problem of generations", used the definition adopted by Heberle, namely, that a generation consisted "of contemporaries of approximately the same age but for whom age is established not by the calendar of years but by a calendar of events and experiences." Heberle concluded that: "A generation is a phenomenon of collective mentality and morality. [The members] of a generation feel themselves linked by a community of standpoints, of beliefs and wishes" (Abrams 1982: 258). But the identification of people as belonging to a particular generation is a complex process. Abrams himself points out that the cut-off points between generations are often obscure and may develop only gradually as part of a long historical process. And this point has been further developed by the American historian Achenbaum (1986), who suggests that the meaning of the term "generation" is "both fuzzy and arbitrary" (Achenbaum 1986: 93). He argues:

> Less clear cut than the distinction between parent and child, the term may refer with equal plausibility to all people between certain ages, to progenitors of any age (as opposed to their progeny), and/or to people who lived through a monumental experience such as the great Depression. The very ambiguity of meaning makes it hard to know who is precisely included or excluded in such a definition. Worse, referring to people as being of a certain generation attributes to them characteristics that they may or may not possess. Who, after all, is a member of the "gypped generation"? Where and how does one draw the line: on the basis of age? birth order? income? expectations? (Achenbaum 1986: 93–4)

This last point is of fundamental importance and was central to the position adopted by Mannheim (1952) in his essay "The problem of generations". Contrary to much of the present speculation about the possible behaviour of generations, Mannheim noted that the characteristic of what he termed "generational units" was that their location and effectiveness in social systems could not be explained adequately on the basis of age alone. Following this, Abrams writes that:

444

Age is a necessary but not a sufficient condition for their existence. Other factors such as class, religion, race, occupation, institutional setting, in short all the conventional categories of social-structural analysis, must be introduced to explain their unique ability to make something of historical experiences. In other words, the study of generations brings to light consequential differentiations within generations as well as between them. Far from exempting us from the study of social structure any attempt to grapple with the problem of the historical formation of identity forces us in just that direction. The emergence of generation units and their capacity or inability to reconstruct identity can only be explained in those terms. Here as elsewhere historical sociology means more work, not less. (Abrams 1982: 261–2)

This analysis does help explain some puzzling features of the way generations behave. For example, reference has been to the argument that there is a growing possibility of the old mobilizing against the interests of the young, and the young threatening to break their part of the generational contract (Thomson 1989). In reality, the evidence for both of these is difficult to find. Wallace et al. (1991) review the former in the American context, suggesting that although older people have been able to influence particular areas of policy and legislation, they have not achieved any enduring pattern of power comparable to that of business or other groups with more focused policy agendas. Wallace et al. (1991) highlight factors that could limit the possibility of a unified movement of older people (see also Binstock 1991).

Within a strong capitalist system, the power of the wealthy and big business will continue to take precedence over the power of the elderly. Most importantly, improvements in the lives of the aged will continue to affect classes differently. For example, elders with secure pensions and investments increasingly have the choice of retiring early or working indefinitely. At the same time, low income workers may be increasingly compelled to continue to work through late life because of financial need or to retire early against their will because of ill health. Consequently, the interests of the aged as a group will continue to be subordinated to class interests and "senior power" will play a secondary role in shaping public policy. (Wallace et al. 1991: 111)

The British case is especially interesting in terms of the welfare generations perspective. Despite the poverty of British pensioners and the government-led campaign against state pensions during the 1980s (Walker 1993a), the voting record of older people in the 1992 election hardly suggested a pattern of militancy on the part of the elderly people; indeed, quite the reverse. Labour raised hopes of a "demographic boost" to their chances with the promise of an immediate pensions increase on election and that future rises would once again be pegged to average wage as well as price rises (whichever rose faster). In fact, the Conservative vote among pensioners hardened – Conservative support among women aged 65 and over (one of the poorest groups) actually increased by 6 per cent in the period between the 1987 and 1992 election (*Sunday Times* 12 April 1992). This might be explained in generational equity terms on the basis that a Conservative government would give succour to the deserving old as opposed to the undeserving young. But the argument is tenuous and there is almost certainly a range of factors lying behind this result. For example, it would appear that among men aged 25–34 the Conservative vote remained remarkably steady – 41 per cent voting Conservative in 1987; 40 per cent in 1992. This suggests, as indicated earlier, that age may be less important than a range of social factors (such as home ownership, social class, membership of a trade union) in interpreting voter behaviour (Walker 1986).

More generally, it is difficult to sustain the view that the 1980s was a clear demonstration of the welfare generation rewarding itself at the expense of others. In fact, in key areas such as jobs, income, and service provision, the evidence suggests considerable inroads were made during the 1980s into the welfare of the old – precisely at a point where they should have been reaping maximum gains. Older workers experienced greater job losses in this decade than any other age group, and this has almost certainly meant extended years in poverty for a significant proportion (Walker 1993a).

In terms of income, the defining characteristic of the 1980s was the declining value of the state pension: relative to average (disposable) incomes it reached a peak of 46.5 per cent in 1983, and by 1992 was lower than it had been in 1948. By 1993 the state pension was worth about 15 per cent of average gross male earnings, lower than at any time since 1971 (Hills 1993). In fact, the most significant feature of the 1980s was not the disparity of incomes between young and old but the growth in inequalities within the older population (Phillipson

1993), a trend that is likely to reduce further the possibility of unified action by the old against the young.

The 1980s were also important for the extended debate on community care, and the respective merits of home-based and residential care. However, it is difficult to see this area as an example of senior power in action. Indeed, what is significant is how little influence older people (or organizations acting on their behalf) had on legislation such as the National Health Service and Community Care Act 1990. On the contrary, this Act may be seen as an attempt to control the demands of the welfare generation, first, through the "marketization" of health and social care (Walker 1993b); secondly, through shifting the burden of care from the formal to the informal sector, with the welfare generation now taking up much of the strain in terms of the provision of personal and social care (Phillipson 1992).

Finally, there is no clear evidence for the young or young middle age rising in protest either against "the crushing of youthful expectations" (Thomson 1989: 53) or the burden of heavy taxation. In the case of Britain, large-scale data sets such as those in the regular series on British Social Attitudes, which have asked the public about priorities for social spending, are consistent in showing a high level of support (across all age groups) for spending on the core welfare services (Taylor-Gooby 1987, 1991). The 1990 survey confirmed the high level of support for "much more" government spending in key areas such as health, welfare and education. Rather than a revolt against taxation, the evidence would suggest increased willingness to pay taxes to support an ageing population – confirmation it would appear of a continuing belief rather than rejection of the intergenerational contract.

The argument from Neugarten and Neugarten (1986) is significant here.

> Some young people now believe they will not enjoy as high a material standard of living as their parents, and some point to the federal budget deficits and to demographic changes to support their assertions that they will not receive as much in Social Security benefits when they grow old. But there is no evidence that young people are blaming old people for what they perceive as this deplorable state of affairs. (Neugarten and Neugarten 1986: 43–4)

The future of the generational contract

If there is limited evidence for open conflict between generations, is it possible to turn the argument around and suggest, instead, that there are signs of mutual interest and solidarity between age groups? The research literature provides at least two examples: one conceptual, and the other empirical. The former starts from the premise that it is more helpful to see generational relations from the standpoint of the life-course as a whole, rather than from a single moment in time (in research terms, taking a longitudinal as opposed to cross-sectional view). This point has been developed by Daniels (1988, 1991) in his concept of the "prudential life-span account". This approach allows the development of guidelines for distribution and redistribution between the life-stages under the condition that all individuals can expect the same treatment over their life-course. In the long run, not only would immediate inequalities be compensated, but also the "prudent" allocation of resources over the life-span would maximize general well-being. Daniels summarizes his perspective in the following terms:

> . . . it tells us we should not think of age groups as competing with each other, but as sharing a whole life. We want to make that life go as well as possible, and we must therefore make the appropriate decisions about what needs it is most important to meet at each stage of life. If we do this prudently, we will learn how fair it is to treat each age group. Instead of focusing on competition, we have a unifying perspective or vision. (Daniels 1991: 238)

This view is matched, it might be argued, in research on how families behave towards each other. The evidence here is that there is giving and receiving throughout the life-course: both within and across generations. Cheal (1987), for example, notes that within the system of family transfers, older people are not solely, or even largely, the recipients of economic resources. He reviews American research in the 1980s which shows that in fact older people are notable providers of resources for others (to younger generations especially). Cheal comments: "It is the propensity of the elderly to give, rather than their necessity to receive, that requires sociological explanation at this time" (Cheal 1987: 141).

216

In Britain, the work of Finch and Mason (1993) has suggested that it is not so much that "experiences of giving and receiving help within families were common experiences (though many of them were) but that they were treated as unremarkable experiences by many people who talked with us" (Finch & Mason 1993, see also Qureshi & Walker 1989).

As indicated in the introduction to this volume, other evidence suggests that integrative forces may be at work, identifying points of mutual interest across generations. Hagestad (1986) puts this in the following way (see also Jerrome 1993b):

> There is little doubt that altered mortality and fertility patterns have created a new climate for the building and maintenance of family relationships. Historians and demographers have suggested that under conditions of high mortality, people were reluctant to form strong attachments to particular individuals, knowing that such ties could not be counted upon to endure. Instead, they invested in the security of the family as a group. Today, most people not only take long-term family bonds for granted and invest accordingly in them, but because of reduced fertility rates, there are also fewer individuals within each generation to invest in. As a result, intergenerational relationships are not only more extensive now, but they may also have become more intensive. Such "intensification of family life" may have gained even further momentum because of the weakening ties between family and community. (Hagestad 1986: 143–4)

These are all positive views as to how generations may gain the benefit of working with each other, taking a long-term view of the compensations from supporting an individual, group or cohort now, in return for receiving support at a later stage. This may sound idealistic, but it might well be argued that this was roughly how society came to reconstruct itself given the reality of population ageing in the postwar period. For a time at least (and even though expressed in often ageist and barely adequate provision), the response to ageing was viewed in public (i.e. intergenerational) terms. The subsequent break with the generational contract was not the result of conflict between generations. Instead it arose from changes (and conflict) at the level of the state as to how this population change should be assimilated.

From an early stage, the language of the Thatcher government in the 1980s was that of "talking-up" the possibility of conflict, suggesting that workers were "reconsidering" how much they should pay in taxes to support pensioners (Phillipson 1990). The value of this approach – for the Conservative government – was that it reinforced the goal of shifting responsibility and perceptions of ageing as a public/life-course issue, to a private/life-stage problem. People had now to think of their own old age rather than that of others (or other generations), and accept that they must rely upon a different kind of welfare. The implications of this is that if there is conflict over the generational contract, it is of a different kind than that envisaged in the worker versus pensioner perspective. The conflict, it might be argued, is between different types of agencies, and different types of ideas. The agency of the state, on the one hand, and the agency of the family, on the other. The view of the aged as public burden, on the one hand, and the view of the aged as a public benefit, on the other. The view of an ageing population as a sign of exhaustion and decline, on the one hand, and view of ageing as a social achievement, on the other. The historical dualism in social images of ageing – between positive and negative perspectives – has swung backwards and forward in the post-war period. We now have to consider ways of restoring a more hopeful future: to seek ways of challenging the current impasse.

Conclusion: towards a new generational politics

In the 1980s and early 1990s the balance swung towards expressing doubts about the benefits of an ageing population. Despite the radical critique offered by the political economy of ageing (Minkler & Estes 1991, Myles & Quadagno 1992), and the activities of groups of older people themselves, the problems of ageing and the welfare state became a dominant theme. In the second half of the 1990s, it is clear that we need a period of renewal in terms of generational politics. The basis for this will come from recognizing that presenting social issues in terms of young versus old does not offer a viable way forward – in the key area of economic and social policy. As Heclo (1989) observes:

> In an already fragmented society such a framework would be especially unconstructive. It would divert attention from dis-

parities and unmet needs within age groups. It would help divide constituencies that often have a common stake. Above all, a politics of young versus old would reinforce an already strong tendency . . . to define social welfare in terms of a competitive struggle for scarce resources and to ignore shared needs occurring in everyone's life-cycle. (Heclo 1989: 387)

Recognition that we are constructing a different type of life-course may also help form the basis for a new generational politics. Here, the worker versus pensioner perspective is especially unhelpful in that it ignores fundamental changes to the distribution of labour through the life-course. The labels "worker" and "pensioner" are less easy to define when the stages that separate them are undergoing change. For many (mostly male) workers the predictability of continuous employment is being replaced by insecurity in middle and later life – an experience shared with the majority of women workers (Itzin & Phillipson 1993). These changes may be seen as part of the reconstruction of middle and old age or the "modernization of ageing" as defined by Featherstone & Hepworth (1988). The social trends here include: a blurring of the boundaries between different stages of the life-course; the growth of different work categories and statuses in between full-time work and complete retirement; and the convergence of male and female employment trends (Laczko & Phillipson 1991).

These trends suggest that a new type of language is necessary for describing relations between generations in general, and workers and pensioners in particular. The language here would stress the interdependency of generations facing radical changes to their traditional social and economic foundations. We are entering a postmodern life-course, one in which individual needs and abilities are no longer entirely subordinate to chronological boundaries and bureaucratic mechanisms (Cole 1992). If the concept of generations has traditionally been elusive and arbitrary, how much more so in a world where the institutions of work and family are being redefined and reshaped.

If we are to take the idea of renewal seriously, the response should not be one of retreat and privatization. Rather, we should acknowledge ageing as a public concern shared equally across the life-course. Above all, we should not "offload" the responsibilities for an ageing population to particular generations or cohorts – whether old, young or middle aged. Ageing is an issue *for* generations, but it is also a question to be *solved* with generations. The role of the state and key economic and social institutions will be central in managing an ageing population. Responsibility for this cannot be put aside in the task of developing appropriate policies for the twenty-first century.

Notes

1. For reviews of the generational equity debate, as viewed from both sides of the Atlantic, see especially Binney & Estes 1988, Walker 1990a, Minkler & Robertson 1991, Phillipson 1991, Johnson & Falkingham 1992.
2. This chapter draws on material gathered whilst the author was in receipt of a research award, from the University of Keele, which enabled him to have an extended period of study in the USA. Particular thanks are due to the Florida Policy on Aging Exchange Centre at the University of South Florida, Tampa, which provided considerable help and support during the author's three month stay in the USA.

Bibliography

Abrams, P. 1978. *Neighbourhood care and social policy*. Berkhamsted: Volunteer Centre.

Abrams, P. 1982. *Historical sociology*. Shepton Mallet: Open Books,

Achenbaum, W. A. 1974. The obsolescence of old age. *Journal of Social History* 8(Fall), 40–52.

Achenbaum, W. A. 1978. *Old age in the new land*. Baltimore, Md: Johns Hopkins University Press.

Achenbaum, W. A. 1986. The meaning of risks, rights, and responsibility in aging America. In *What does it mean to grow old?*, T. Cole & S. Gadow (eds), 92–103. Durham, NC: Duke University Press.

Achenbaum, W. A. 1989. Public pensions as intergenerational transfers in the United States. See Johnson et al. (1989), 113–36.

Acock, A. C. 1984. Parents and their children: the study of intergenerational difference. *Sociology and Social Research* 68(2), 151–71.

Allatt, P. & S. Yeandle 1986. "It's not fair, is it?" Youth unemployment, family relationships & the social contract. In *The experience of unemployment*, S. Allen, A. Watson, K. Purcell, S. Wood (eds), 104–21. London: Macmillan.

Allen, K. 1989. *Single women/family ties*. Beverly Hills, Calif.: Sage.

Anderson, M. 1977. The impact on the family relationship of the elderly of changes since Victorian times in governmental income maintenance. In *Family bureaucracy and the elderly*, E. Shanas & M. Sussman (eds), 36–59. Durham, NC: Duke University Press.

Anderson, M. 1979. The relevance of family history. In *The sociology of the family: new directions for Britain*, C. Harris (ed.). Sociological Review Monograph 28: 118–40.

Anderson, M. 1985. The emergence of the modern life-cycle. *Social History* 10(1), 69–87.

Anderson, M. 1990. Households, families and individuals: some preliminary results from the national sample from the 1851 census of Great Britain. *Continuity and Change* 3, 421–38.

Arber, S. & N. Gilbert 1989. Transitions in later life: gender, life-course and care of the elderly. In *Becoming and being old*, B. Bytheway, T. Kiel. P. Allatt, A. Bryman (eds), 72–92. London: Sage.

Arber, S. & J. Ginn 1990. The meaning of informal care: gender and the contribution of elderly people. *Ageing and Society* **10**(4), 429–54.

Arber, S. & J. Ginn 1991. *Gender and later life: a sociological analysis of resources and constraints*. London: Sage.

Arber, S., N. Gilbert, M. Evandrou 1988. Gender, household composition and receipt of domiciliary services by the elderly disabled. *Journal of Social Policy* **17**(2), 153–76.

Ascherson, N. 1986. London's new class: the great cash-in. *Observer*.

Atkin, K. 1991. Community care in a multi-racial society: incorporating the user view. *Policy and Politics* **19**(3), 159–66.

Atkin, K. 1992. Black carers: the forgotten people. *Nursing the Elderly* (March/April), 8–9.

Atkin, K. & J. Rollings 1992. Informal care in Asian and Afro/Caribbean communities: a literature review. *British Journal of Social Work* **22**, 405–18.

Atkinson, A. B. 1978. *Distribution of personal wealth in Britain*. Oxford: Clarendon.

Atkinson, A. B., J. P. Gordon, A. Harrison 1989. Trends in the shares of top wealth holders in Britain, 1923–1981. *Oxford Bulletin of Economics and Statistics* **51**(3), 315–32.

Attias-Donfut, C. 1988. *Sociologie des générations*. Paris: Presses Universitaires de France.

Baltes, P. B., J. Smith, U. M. Standinger 1992. Wisdom and successful aging. In *Nebraska Symposium on Motivation*, T. B. Sonderegger (ed.) **39**, 123–67. Lincoln, Nebr.: University of Nebraska Press.

Bamford, C. 1993. The transitions of later life: learning from the past. *Journal of Educational Gerontology* **8**(1), 7–17.

Bamford, C. 1994. *Grandparents' lives: men and women in later life*. Edinburgh: Age Concern Scotland.

Barrett, M. 1980. *Women's oppression today*. London: Verso.

Barrett, M. & M. McIntosh 1982. *The anti-social family*. London: Verso.

Bebbington, A. 1988. The expectation of life without disability in England and Wales. *Social Science and Medicine* **27**(4), 321–7.

Becker, H. A. 1987. *Generations and social inequality*. Utrecht: Uiteverij Tanvan Arkel.

Bell, C. 1968. *Middle class families*. London: Routledge & Kegan Paul.

Bengston, V. 1987. Parenting, grandparenting and intergenerational continuity. In *Parenting across the lifespan: biosocial dimensions*, J. B. Lancaster, J. Altman, A. S. Rossi, L. R. Sherrod (eds), 435–56. Berlin and New York: Aldine de Gruyter.

Bengston, V. 1989. The problem of generations: age group contrasts, continuities and social change. In *The course of adult life*, V. Bengston & K. Shaife (eds), 25–54. New York: Springer.

Bengston, V. 1993. Is the "contract across generations" changing? Effects of population ageing on obligations and expectations across age groups. See Bengston & Achenbaum (1993), 3–24.

Bengston, V. & W. A. Achenbaum (eds) 1993. *The changing contract across generations*. New York: Aldine.

Bengston, V. L. & J. F. Robertson 1985. *Grandparenthood*. Beverly Hills, Calif.: Sage.

Bengston, V. L., N. E. Cutler, D. J. Mangen, V. W. Marshall 1985. Generations, cohorts, and relations between age groups. In *Handbook of ageing and the social services*, R. Binstock & E. Shanas (eds), 304–38. New York: Van Nostrand Reinhold.

Bengston, V. L., G. Marti, R. E. L. Roberts 1991. Age group relations: generational equity and inequity. In *Parent–child relations across the lifespan*, K. Pillemer & K. McCartney (eds), 253–78. Hillsdale, NJ: Lawrence Erlbaum

Beveridge, W. 1942. *Social insurance and allied services*. London: HMSO.

Bhaduri, R. & R. Wright 1990. *Social services and members of black and ethnic minority communities*. London Social Services Inspectorate, Department of Health.

Binney, E. A. & C. L. Estes 1988. The retreat of the state and its transfer of responsibility: the intergenerational war. *International Journal of Health Services* **18**(1), 83–96.

Binstock, R. 1983. The aged as scapegoat. *The Gerontologist* **23**(4), 136–43.

Binstock, R. 1991. Aging, politics, and public policy. In *Growing old in America*, B. Hess & E. Markson (eds), 325–40. New Brunswick, NJ: Transaction.

Binstock, R. 1994. Transcending intergenerational equity. See Marmor et al. (1994), 155–85.

Blackburn, R. & J. Jarman 1993. Changing inequalities in access to British universities. *Oxford Review of Education* **19**(2), 197–215.

Blakemore, K. 1983. Ageing in the inner city: a comparison of old blacks and whites. In *Ageing in modern society*, D. Jerrome (ed.), 81–103. London: Croom Helm.

Booth, C. 1894. *The aged poor in England and Wales*. London: Macmillan.

Bornat, J., C. Phillipson, S. Ward 1985. *A manifesto for old age*. London: Pluto Press.

Brody, E. 1981. "Women in the middle" and family help to older people. *The Gerontologist* **21**(15), 471–9.

Brody, E. 1985. Parent care as a normative family stress. *The Gerontologist* **25**(1), 19–25.

Butt, J., P. Gorbach, B. Ahmad 1991. *Equally fair?* London: Race Equality Unit, National Institute for Social Work.

Callahan, D. 1987. *Setting limits: medical goals in an aging society*. New York: Simon & Schuster.

Cameron, E., H. Evers, F. Badger, K. Atkin 1989. Black old women, disability and health carers. In *Growing old in the twentieth century*, M. Jefferys (ed.), 230–48. London: Routledge.

Carlesworth, A., D. Wilkin, A. Durie 1984. *Carers and services: a comparison of men and women providing services to dependent elderly people*. Manchester: Equal Opportunities Commission.

Carnegie Inquiry into the Third Age 1993. *Life, work and livelihood in the Third Age*, Final Report. Dunfermline: Carnegie UK Trusts.

Casey, B. & F. Laczko 1989. Early retired or long-term unemployed? The situation of non-working men aged 55–64 from 1979 to 1986. *Work, Employment and Society* 3(4): 509–26.

Central Statistics Office, Dublin 1983. *Census of Population of Ireland 1979*. Dublin: Central Statistics Office.

Cheal, D. 1987. Intergenerational transfers and life course management: towards a socio-economic perspective. In *Re-thinking the life-cycle*, A. Bryman, P. Allatt, T. Keill (eds), 55–73. London: Macmillan.

Checkland, S. G. & E. O. A. Checkland (eds) 1974. *The Poor Law Report of 1834*. Harmondsworth: Penguin.

Cherlin, A. & F. Furstenberg 1985. Style and strategies of grandparenting. See Bengston & Robertson (1985), 170–92.

Cicirelli, V. 1983. Adult children and their elderly parents. In *Family relationships in later life*, T. Brubaker (ed.), 31–46. Beverly Hills, Calif.: Sage.

Clark, R. & J. Spengler 1980. *The economics of individual and population aging*. Cambridge: Cambridge University Press.

Cohen, C. (ed.) 1993. *Justice across generations*. Washington, DC: American Association of Retired Persons.

Cole, T. R. 1992. *The journey of life: a cultural history of aging in America*. Cambridge: Cambridge University Press.

Coleman, P. & A. McCulloch 1985. The study of psychosocial change in later life. In *Lifespan and change in a gerontological perspective*, J. Munnichs et al. (eds), 239–55. New York: Springer.

Commission of the European Communities 1990. *Proposal for a Council decision on community actions for the elderly*, Com (90) 80, 24 April, Luxembourg.

Commission of the European Communities 1994. *Social protection in Europe*. Luxembourg: Office for Official Publications of the European Communities.

Dalley, G. 1988. *Ideologies of caring*. London: Macmillan.

Daniels, N. 1988. *Am I my parents' keeper?* Oxford and New York: Oxford University Press.

Daniels, N. 1991. A lifespan approach to health care. In *Aging and ethics*, A. Jecker (ed.), 227–46. Princeton, NJ: Humana Press.

Dannefer, D. 1988. What's in a name? An account of the neglect of variability in the study of aging. In *Emergent theories of aging*, J. Birren & V. Bengston (eds), 356–84. New York: Springer.

Davidoff, L. & C. Hall 1987. *Family fortunes: men and women of the English middle class*. London: Hutchinson.

Davies, B. & D. Challis 1986. *Matching resources for needs in community care*. Aldershot: Gower.

Davies, J. A. 1986. British and American attitudes: similarities and contrasts. In *British social attitudes*, R. Jowell, S. Witherspoon, L. Brook (eds), 89–114. Aldershot: Gower.

Davis, E. P. & I. D. Saville 1982. Mortgage lending and the housing market. *Bank of England Quarterly Bulletin* (September), 390–98.

Davis Smith, J. 1992. *Volunteering: widening horizons in the third age*. Report for the Carnegie Inquiry into the Third Age, London.

Department of Employment 1992. *Labour Force Survey 1990*. London: HMSO.

Department of Trade and Industry 1995. *Competitiveness: forging ahead*, Cm 2867. London: HMSO.

DH/DSS/Scottish and Welsh Offices 1989. *Caring for people: community care in the next decade and beyond*. Govt White Paper. London: HMSO.

DHSS 1981. *Growing older*. Govt White Paper. London: HMSO.

DHSS 1985a. *Reform of social security*, Cmnd 9517. London: HMSO.

DHSS 1985b. *Reform of social security: programme for change*. London: HMSO.

Donzelot, J. 1979. *The policing of families*. London: Hutchinson.

Easterlin, R. A. 1978. What will 1984 be like? Socio-economic implications of recent shifts in age structure. *Demography* **15**, 397–432.

Engels, F. 1884. *The origins of the family, private property and the state*. Republished 1985. Harmondsworth: Penguin.

Equal Opportunities Commission 1980. *The experience of caring for elderly and handicapped dependents*. Manchester: EOC.

Ermisch, J. 1990. *Fewer babies, longer lives: policy implications of current demographic trends*. York: Joseph Rowntree Foundation.

Estes, C. 1992. The Reagan legacy: privatization, the welfare state, and ageing in the 1990s. See Myles & Quadagno (1992), 59–83.

Estes, C. L., J. Swan, L. Gerard 1982. Dominant and competing paradigms in gerontology: towards a political economy of ageing. *Ageing and Society* **2**(2), 69–85.

Falkingham, J. & J. Hills (eds) 1995. *The dynamic of welfare: social policy and the life-cycle*. Hemel Hempstead: Harvester Wheatsheaf.

Featherstone, M. & M. Hepworth 1988. Ageing and old age: reflections on the postmodern lifecourse. In *Being and becoming old*, B. Bytheway, T. Keil, P. Allatt, A. Bryman (eds), 143–57. London: Sage.

Finch, J. 1987. Whose responsibility? Women and the future of family care. In *Informal care tomorrow*, I. Allen (ed.), 34–48. London: Policy Studies Institute.

Finch, J. 1989. *Family obligations and social change*. Oxford: Polity Press.

Finch, J. 1990. The politics of community care in Britain. In *Gender and caring: work and welfare in Britain and Scandinavia*, C. Ungerson (ed.), 119–40. Hemel Hempstead: Harvester Wheatsheaf.

Finch, J. & D. Groves 1980. Community care and the family: a case for equal opportunities? *Journal of Social Policy* **9**(4), 487–514.

Finch, J. & D. Groves (eds) 1983. *A labour of love: women, work and caring*. London: Routledge & Kegan Paul.

Finch, J. & J. Mason 1990. Filial obligations and kin support for elderly people. *Ageing and Society* **10**(2), 151–76.

Finch, J. & J. Mason 1991. Obligations of kinship in contemporary Britain. *British Journal of Sociology* **42**(3), 344–67.

Finch, J. & J. Mason 1993. *Negotiating family responsibilities*. London: Routledge.

Finch, J. & L. Wallis 1993. Inheritance, care bargains and elderly people's relationships with their children. In *Health and community care: UK and international perspectives*, D. Challis & B. Davies (eds), 64–82. Aldershot: Gower.

Finch, J., L. Hayes, J. Mason, J. Masson, L. Wallis 1995. *Wills inheritance and the family*. Oxford: Oxford University Press.

Fiske, M. & D. Chiriboga 1985. The interweaving of societal and personal change in adulthood. In *Lifespan and change in a gerontological perspective*, J. Munnichs et al. (eds), 117–85. New York: Springer.

Foote, D. 1982. *Canada's population outlook: demographic futures and economic challenges*. Ottawa: Canadian Institute for Economic Policy.

Forrest, R. & A. Murie 1989. Differential accumulation: wealth, inheritance and housing policy. *Policy and Politics* **17**(1), 25–39.

Forster, M. 1989. *Have the men had enough?* Harmondsworth: Penguin.

Francis, D. 1984. *Will you still need me, will you still feed me, when I'm 84?* Bloomington, Ind.: Indiana University Press.

Friedman, M. & R. Friedman 1980. *Free to choose*. Harmondsworth: Penguin.

Fry, P. S. 1992. A consideration of cognitive factors in the learning and education of older adults. *International Review of Education* **38**(4), 303–26.

Garrett, E. & A. Reid 1994. Satanic mills, pleasant lands: spatial variation in women's work, fertility and infant mortality as viewed from the 1991 census. *Historical Research* **67**, 158–77.

Gavron, H. 1966. *The captive wife*. London: Routledge & Kegan Paul.

Gibson, C. 1990. Widowhood: patterns, problems and choices. In *Aspects of ageing Social Policy Papers 3*, M. Bury & J. Macnicol (eds), 82–103. Royal Holloway and Bedford New College.

Gilhooley, M. 1986. Senile dementia: factors associated with caregivers' preference for institutional care. *British Journal of Medical Psychology* **59**, 165–71.

Gilleard, C., H. Belford, J. Gilleard, J. Whittick, K. Gledhill 1984. Emotional distress amongst supporters of the elderly mentally infirm. *British Journal of Psychiatry* **145**, 172–7.

Glass, J., V. Bengston, C. Dunham 1986. Attitude similarity in 3-generational families: socialization, status inheritance or reciprocal influence. *American Sociological Review* **51**, 685–98.

Glendenning, F. 1983. Ethnic minority elderly people: some issues of social policy. In *Social work and ethnicity*, J. Cheetham (ed.), 122–31. London: Allen & Unwin.

Glendenning, F. 1990. The emergence of educational gerontology. In *Ageing, education and society: readings in educational gerontology*, F. Glendenning & K. Percy (eds). Keele: Association for Educational Gerontology.

Goldscheider, F. 1990. The aging of the gender revolution: what do we know and what do we need to know? *Research on Aging* **12**(4), 531–45.

Gouldner, A. W. 1960. The norm of reciprocity. *American Sociological Review* **25**, 161–78.

Government Actuary 1990. *National Insurance fund: long term financial estimates*, HC(89–90) 582. London: HMSO.

Graebner, W. 1980. *A history of retirement*. New Haven, Conn.: Yale University Press.

Green, H. 1988. *Informal carers*. London: HMSO.

Griffiths, R. 1988. *Agenda for action*. London: HMSO.

Guillemard, A.-M. 1980. *La Vieillesse et l'état*. Paris: Presses Universitaires de France.

Guillemard, A.-M. 1993. Older workers and the labour market. See Walker et al. (1993), 68–99.

Gutmann, D. 1987. *Reclaimed powers*. New York: Basic Books.

Hagestad, G. 1985. Older women in intergenerational relations. In *The physical and mental health of aged women*, M. Haug, A. Ford, M. Shearer (eds), 112–34. New York: Springer.

Hagestad, G. 1986. The family: women and the family as kin-keepers. In *Our aging society*, A. Pifer & L. Bronte (eds), 141–60. Ontario: Norton.

Hagestad, G. 1987. Parent–child relations in later life: trends and gaps in past research. In *Parenting across the lifespan: biosocial dimensions*, J. B. Lancaster, A. S. Reiss, L. R. Sherrod (eds), 405–33. Berlin and New York: Aldine de Gruyter.

Hagestad, G. 1988. Demographic change and the life course: some emerging trends in the family realm. *Family Relations* 37, 405–10.

Hamnett, C. 1991. A nation of inheritors? Housing inheritance, wealth and inequality in Britain. *Journal of Social Policy* 20(4), 509–36.

Hamnett, C. & B. Mullings 1992a. The distribution of public and private residential homes for elderly persons in England and Wales. *Area* 24(2), 130–44.

Hamnett, C. & B. Mullings 1992b. A new consumption cleavage? The case of residential care for the elderly. *Environment and Planning A*, 24, 807–20.

Hamnett, C. & P. Williams 1993. Housing wealth and inheritance. In *Housing finance and subsidies in Britain*, D. McLennan & K. Gibb (eds), 137–62. Aldershot: Avebury.

Hamnett, C., M. Harmer, P. Williams 1991. *Safe as houses: housing inheritance in Britain*. London: Paul Chapman.

Hansard 1989. Weekly Hansard 1493(10–14 July). London: HMSO.

Harbury, C. 1962. Inheritance and the distribution of personal wealth in Britain. *Economic Journal* 72, 854–68.

Harbury, C & D. Hitchens 1979. *Inheritance and wealth inequality in Britain*. London: Allen & Unwin.

Harper, S. 1992. Caring for China's ageing population: the residential option – a case study of Shanghai. *Ageing and Society* 12(?), 157–84.

Harion, H 1990. *The Himba people*. London: Routledge.

Hazelzet, K. 1990. *De levenstrap*. Zwolle: Uitgeverij Catena.

Heclo, H. 1989. Generational politics. In *The vulnerable*, T. Smeeding & B. Torrey (eds), 381–441. Washington, DC: Urban Institute Press.

Henwood, M. 1992. *Through a glass darkly: community care and elderly people*. London: King's Fund Institute.

Hills, J. 1992. Does Britain have a "welfare generation"? An empirical analysis of intergenerational equity, Welfare State Programme Discussion Paper WSP/76. London: London School of Economics.

Hills, J. 1993. *The future of welfare: a guide to the debate*. York: Joseph Rowntree Foundation.

Hills, J. 1995. The welfare state and redistribution between generations. See Falkingham & Hills (1995), 100–128.

Hinrichs, K. 1991. Insecurity regarding social security: public pensions and demographic change in Germany. In *Inter-generational rivalries*, J. Guillemin & I. Horowitz (eds). New York: Transaction.

HM Treasury 1993. *Public expenditure analyses to 1995-96*, Cm 2219. London: HMSO.

Hobman, D. (ed.) 1993. *Uniting generations*. London: Age Concern England.

Holmans, A. 1986. *Flows of funds associated with house purchase for owner occupation in the United Kingdom 1977–1984 and equity withdrawal from house purchase finance*. Government Economic Service Working Paper 92, January, London.

Holmans, A. 1990. *House prices: changes through time at the national and sub-national level*. Government Economic Service Working Paper 110, December, London.

Holmans, A. 1991. *Estimates of housing equity withdrawal by owner occupiers in the United Kingdom 1970 to 1990*. Government Economic Service Working Paper 116, November, London.

Holstein, M. 1993. Women's lives, women's work: productivity, gender and aging. In *Achieving a productive ageing society*, S. A. Bass, F. Caro, Y-P. Chen (eds), 235–48. Westport, Conn.: Greenwood.

Homer, P. & M. Holstein (eds) 1990. *A good old age: the paradox of setting limits*. New York: Touchstone.

Hoyes, L., R. Means, J. Le Grand 1992. *Made to measure: performance measurement and community care*. School for Advanced Urban Studies, University of Bristol.

Inland Revenue 1986. *Inland Revenue Statistics*. London: HMSO.

Inland Revenue 1990. *Inland Revenue Statistics*. London: HMSO.

Inland Revenue 1991. *Inland Revenue Statistics*. London: HMSO.

Inland Revenue 1993. *Inland Revenue Statistics*. London: HMSO.

Itzin, C. & C. Phillipson 1993. *Age barriers at work*. Solihull: METRA, Metropolitan Authorities Recruitment Agency.

James, N. 1993. Inheritance: all our futures. *Lloyds Bank Economic Bulletin* 176 (August).

Jerrome, D. 1990. Intimate relationships. In *Ageing in society: an introduction to social gerontology*, J. Bond & P. Coleman (eds), 181–208. London: Sage.

Jerrome, D. 1991. Social bonds in later life. *Reviews in Clinical Gerontology* 1, 297–306.

Jerrome, D. 1992. *Good company: an anthropological study of old people in groups*. Edinburgh: Edinburgh University Press.

Jerrome, D. 1993a. Intimacy and sexuality amongst older women. In *Women come of age*, M. Bernard and K. Meade (eds), 85–105. London: Edward Arnold.

Jerrome, D. 1993b. Intimate relationships. In *Ageing and society*, J. Bond, P. Coleman, S. Peace (eds), 226–54. London: Sage.

Jerrome, D. 1994a. Time, change and continuity in family life. *Ageing and Society* 14(1), 1–27.

Jerrome, D. 1994b. Family estrangement: parents and children who lose touch. *Journal of Family Therapy* 16(4), 241–58.

Jerrome, D. 1996. *The family in time and space*. Occasional paper. Mass Observation Archive, University of Sussex.

Johanson, S. R. (1991) Welfare, mortality and gender: continuity and change in explanations for male/female mortality differences over three centuries. *Continuity and Change* 6, 135–77.

Johnson, P. & J. Falkingham 1988a. *Intergenerational transfers and public expenditure on the elderly in modern Britain*. London: Centre for Economic Policy Research.

Johnson, P. & J. Falkingham 1988b. Intergenerational transfers and public expenditure on the elderly in modern Britain. *Ageing and Society* 8, 129–46.

Johnson, P. & J. Falkingham 1992. *Ageing and economic welfare*. London: Sage.

Johnson, P., C. Conrad, D. Thomson (eds) 1989. *Workers versus pensioners: intergenerational justice in an ageing world*. Manchester: Manchester University Press in association with the Centre for Economic Policy Research.

Jones, J. 1988. Ageing and generational equity: an American perspective Paper given at an international seminar on the ageing of the population, Futuribles International, Paris, mimeo.

Kington, E., B. Hirshorn, J. Cornman 1986. *Ties that bind: the interdependence of generations in an ageing society*. Maryland: Seven Locks Press.

Kohli, M. 1993. Public solidarity between generations: historical and comparative elements. Paper presented at Conference on Older people and solidarity between generations, November, Paris.

Kohli, M., M. Rein, A.-M. Guillemard, H. Gunsteren (eds) 1991. *Time for retirement*. Cambridge: Cambridge University Press.

Kornhaber, A. 1985. Grandparenthood and the new social contract. See Bengston & Robertson (1985), 159–72.

Kotlikoff, T. J 1992. *Generational accounting: knowing who pays, and when, for what we spend*. New York: Free Press.

Kreps, J. 1977. Intergenerational transfers and the bureaucracy. In *Family bureaucracy and the elderly*, E. Shanas & M. Sussman (eds). Durham, NC: Duke University Press.

Kuhn, M. 1991. *No stone unturned*. New York: Random House.

Laczko, F. & C. Phillipson 1990. Defending the right to work. In *Age: the unrecognised discrimination*, E. McEwan (ed.). London: ACE Books.

Laczko, F. & C. Phillipson 1991. *Changing work and retirement: social policy and the older worker*. Milton Keynes: Open University Press

Land, H. 1978. Who cares for the family? *Journal of Social Policy* 7(3), 357–84.

Land, H. & H. Rose 1985. Compulsory altruism or an altruistic society for all? In *In defence of welfare*, P. Bean et al. (eds), 74–98. London: Tavistock.

Langan, M. & I. Ostner 1991. Gender and welfare. In *Towards a European welfare state?* G. Room (ed.), 127–50. Bristol: School for Advanced Urban Studies.

Laslett, P. 1965. *The world we have lost*. London: Methuen.

Laslett, P. 1989. *A fresh map of life*. London: Weidenfeld & Nicolson.

Laslett, P. & J. Fishkin (eds) 1992a. *Justice between age groups and generations*. New Haven, Conn.: Yale University Press.

Laslett, P. & J. Fishkin 1992b. Introduction: processional justice. See Laslett & Fishkin (1992a), 1–23.

Leather, P. 1990. The potential and implications of home equity release in old age. *Housing Studies* 5(1), 3–13.

Levin, E., I. Sinclair, P. Gorbach 1986. *Families, services and confusion in old age*. London: Allen & Unwin.

Lewis, J. 1993. *Women and social policies in Europe*. Aldershot: Edward Elgar.

Lewis, J. & B. Meredith 1988. *Daughters who care*. London: Routledge.

Lindley, R., R. Wilson, E. Villagomez 1991. *Labour market prospects for the third age*. Warwick: Institute for Employment Research.

Lomax Cook, F. 1990. Congress and the public: convergent and divergent opinions on social security. In *Social security and the budget*, H. J. Aaron (ed.), 79–107. New York: University Press.

Longman, P. 1987. *Born to pay: the politics of aging in America*. Boston, Mass.: Houghton Mifflin.

Lowe, R. 1993. *The welfare state in Britain since 1945*. London: Macmillan.

Macfarlane, A. 1978. *The origins of English individualism: the family, property and social transition*. Oxford: Blackwell.

Mannheim, K. 1952. The problem of generations. *Essays on the sociology of knowledge*. London: Routledge & Kegan Paul.

Marmor, T. R., J. L. Mashaw, P. L. Harvey 1990. *America's misunderstood welfare state*. New York: Basic Books.

Marmor, T., T. Smeeding, V. Green (eds) 1994. *Economic security and intergenerational justice*. Washington, DC: Urban Institute Press.

Marshall, V., C. Rosenthal, J. Dacink 1987. Older parents' expectations for filial support. *Social Justice Research* 1(4), 405–24.

Marshall, V. W., F. Lomax Cook, J. G. Marshall 1993. Conflict over intergenerational equity: rhetoric and reality in a comparative context. See Bengston & Achenbaum (1993), 119–40.

McGoldrick, A. & C. Cooper 1980. Voluntary early retirement: taking the decision. *Employment Gazette* (August).

McKay, S. 1992. *Pensioners' assets*. London: Policy Studies Institute.

Midwinter, E. 1992. *Citizenship: from ageism to participation*. London: Report for the Carnegie Inquiry into the Third Age.

Minkler, M. 1986. "Generational equity" and the new victim blaming: an emerging public policy issue. *International Journal of Health Services* 16(4), 539–51.

Minkler, M. & C. Estes 1991. *Critical perspectives on aging*. New York: Baywood.

Minkler, M. & A. Robertson 1991. The ideology of age/race wars: deconstructing a social problem. *Ageing and Society* 11, 1–23.

Moody, H. 1988. *Abundance of life: human development policies for an aging society*. New York: Columbia University Press.

Moody, H. 1992. Bioethics and aging. In *Handbook of the humanities and aging*, T. Cole, D. Van Tassell, R. Kastenbaum (eds), 395–425. New York: Springer.

Moody, H. R. 1993. A strategy for productive aging: education in later life. In *Achieving a productive ageing society*, S. A. Bass, F. Caro, Y-P. Chen (eds), 221–32. Westport, Conn.: Greenwood.

Morgan Grenfell 1987. Housing inheritance and wealth. *Morgan Grenfell Economic Review* 45 (November).

Morgan Grenfell 1993. Housing inheritance: how much, how soon? Morgan Grenfell Economics. UK *Economic Issues* (July).

Moroney, R. M. 1976. *The family and the state*. London: Longman.

Morris, C. (ed.) 1947. *The journal of Celia Fiennes*. London: Cresset Press.

Morris, L. 1985. Renegotiation of the domestic division of labour in the context of male redundancy. In *New approaches to economic life*, B. Roberts, R.

Finnegan, D. Gallie (eds). Manchester: Manchester University Press.

Mullings, B. & C. Hamnett 1992. Equity release schemes and equity extraction by elderly households in Britain. *Ageing and Society* 12, 413–42.

Munro, M. 1987. Housing, health and inheritance. *Journal of Social Policy* 17(4), 417–36.

Murie, A. & R. Forrest 1980. Wealth, inheritance and housing policy. *Policy and Politics* 8(1), 1–19.

Myerhoff, B. 1978. *Number our days*. New York: Simon & Schuster.

Myles, J. 1983. Conflict, crisis, and the future of old age security. *Millbank Memorial Fund Quarterly* 61(3), 462–72.

Myles, J. 1984. *Old age in the welfare state*. Boston, Mass.: Little Brown.

Myles, J. & J. Quadagno (eds) 1992. *States, labour markets and the future of old-age policy*. Philadelphia, Pa.: Temple University Press.

National Economic Development Office 1989. *Defusing the demographic timebomb*. London: NEDO.

Neugarten, B. & D. Neugarten 1986. Changing meanings of age in the aging society. In *Our aging society: paradox and promise*, A. Pifer & L. Bronte (eds), 33–52. Ontario. Norton.

Nissel, M. & L. Bonnerjea 1982. *Family care of the handicapped elderly: who pays?* London: Policy Studies Institute.

O'Connor, P. 1992. *Friendships between women*. Brighton: Harvester Wheatsheaf.

OECD 1988a. *Reforming public pensions*. Paris: OECD.

OECD 1988b. *Ageing populations: the social policy implications*. Paris: OECD.

OECD 1994. *New orientations for social policy*. Paris: OECD.

Office of Population Censuses and Surveys 1990. *General Household Survey 1988*. London: HMSO.

Office of Population Censuses and Surveys 1993. *National Population Projections 1991-based*, series PP2 18. London: HMSO.

Osako, M. & W. Liu 1986. Intergenerational relations and the aged among Japanese Americans. *Research on Aging* 8(1), 128–55.

Pampel, F, J. Williamson, R. Stryker 1990. Class context and pension response to demographic structure in advanced industrial democracies. *Social Problems* 37(4), 535–50.

Parker, G. 1990. *With due care and attention: a review of research on informal care*. London: Family Policy Studies Centre.

Peterson, D. A. 1983. *Facilitating education for older learners*. London: Jossey Bass.

Phillipson, C. 1982. *Capitalism and the construction of old age*. London: Macmillan.

Phillipson, C. 1990. Inter-generational relations: conflict or consensus in the twenty-first century? *Policy and Politics* 19, 27–36.

Phillipson, C. 1992. Challenging the "spectre of old age": community care for older people in the 1990s. In *Social Policy Review 4*, N. Manning & R. Page (eds), 111–33. Canterbury: Social Policy Association.

Phillipson, C. 1993. Poverty and affluence in old age. In *Poverty, inequality and justice*, A. Sinfield (ed.). Edinburgh: New Waverley Papers, Social Policy Series 6.

Phillipson, C. & A. Walker (eds) 1986. *Ageing and social policy*. Aldershot: Gower.

Pollitt, P. 1991. Senile dementia in the family and the response of male relatives. Paper presented at British Sociological Association Conference, Manchester, March.

Pollitt, P. A., I. Anderson, D. O'Connor 1991. For better or worse: the experience of caring for an elderly dementing spouse. *Ageing and Society* **11**(4), 443–69.

Preston, S. 1984. Children and the elderly: divergent paths for America's dependents. *Demography* **XXI**, 435–57.

Quadagno, J. 1989. Generational equity and the politics of the welfare state. *Politics and Society* **17**(3), 353–76.

Qureshi, H. 1986. Responses to dependency: reciprocity, affect and power in family relationships. In *Dependency and interdependency in old age*, C. Phillipson, M. Bernard, P. Strang (eds), 167–89. London: Croom Helm.

Qureshi, H. & K. Simons 1987. Resources within families: caring for elderly people. In *Give and take in families*, J. Brannen & G. Wilson (eds), 117–35. London: Allen & Unwin.

Qureshi, H. & A. Walker 1989. *The caring relationships: elderly people and their families*. Basingstoke: Macmillan/New York: Temple University Press.

Reday-Mulvey, G. 1990. Work and retirement: future prospects for the baby-boom generation. *Geneva Papers* **55**, 100–13.

Riley, M. W. 1985. Women, men and the lengthening life course. In *Gender and the life course*, A. Rossi (ed.), 333–48. New York: Aldine.

Riley, M. W. 1991. Cohort perspectives. In *The encylopaedia of sociology*, E. F. Borgatta & M. L. Borgatta (eds), 413–18. New York: Macmillan.

Riley, M. W. & J. W. Riley 1993. Connections: kin and cohort. See Bengston & Achenbaum (1993), 169–90.

Riley, M., M. Johnson, A. Foner 1972. *Aging and society* **3**: *a sociology of age stratification*. New York: Russel Sage Foundation.

Robin, J. 1990. The relief of poverty in mid-19th century Colyton. *Rural Society* **1**, 193–218.

Rosenthal, C. 1985. Kinkeeping in the familial division of labour. *Journal of Marriage and the Family* **47**, 965–74.

Rosow, I. 1962. Old age: one moral dilemma of the affluent society. *The Gerontologist* **2**, 182–91.

Royal Commission on Population 1949. *Report*. London: HMSO.

Royal Commission on the Distribution of Income and Wealth 1977. *Third report on the standing reference*, Report 5, Cmnd 6999. London: HMSO.

Royal Commission on the Distribution of Income and Wealth 1978. (Chairman Lord Diamond) *Report*. London: HMSO.

Rubenson, K. 1989. Swedish adult education policy in the 1970s and 1980s. In *The Struggle for democratic education: equality and participation in Sweden*, S. Ball & S. Larsson (eds), 136–55. Lewes: Falmer Press.

Ruggles, S. 1987. *Prolonged connections: the rise of the extended family in 19th century England and America*. Madison, Wis.: University of Wisconsin Press.

Ruoppila, I. 1991. The significance of grandparents for the formation of family relations. In *The psychology of grandparenthood: an international perspective*,

P. K. Smith (ed.), 123–42. London: Routledge.

Saunders, P. 1986. Comment on Dunleavy and Preteceille. *Society and Space* **4**, 155–63.

Schorr, A. 1992. *The personal social services: an outside view*. York: Joseph Rowntree Foundation.

Schuller, T. 1993. A temporal approach to the relationship between education and generation. *Time and Society* **2**(3), 335–51.

Schuller, T. & A. M. Bostyn 1992. *Learning: education, training and information in the third age*, Report for the Carnegie Inquiry into the Third Age, London.

Schultz, J. 1988. *The economics of aging*. Belmont, Calif.: Wadsworth.

Seale, C. 1990. Caring for people who die: the experience of family and friends. *Ageing and Society* **10**(4), 413–28.

Secretary of State for Social Services 1980. Minutes of Evidence to the House of Commons Social Services Committee 22 May, 702–II, London: HMSO.

Shanas, E. & G. Streib (eds) 1965. *Social structure and the family: generational relations*. London: Prentice Hall.

Shanas, E., P. Townsend, D. Wedderburn, H. Friis, P. Milhöj, J. Stehouwer 1968. *Old people in three industrial societies*. London: Routledge & Kegan Paul.

Shirley, I. 1990. New Zealand: the advance of the new right. In *The social effects of free market policies: an international text*, I. Taylor (ed.), 351–90. London: Harvester Wheatsheaf.

Shorter, E. 1977. *The making of the modern family*. Glasgow: Fontana/Collins.

Siim, B. 1990. Women and the welfare state: between private and public dependence. A comparative approach to care work in Denmark and Britain. In *Gender and caring: work and welfare in Britain and Scandinavia*, C. Ungerson (ed.), 80–109. Hemel Hempstead: Harvester Wheatsheaf.

Social Trends 1993. Central Statistical Office, London: HMSO.

Spitze, G. & J. Logan 1989. Gender differences in family support: is there a payoff? *The Gerontologist* **29**(1), 108–13.

Spitze, G. & L. Miner 1992. Gender differences in adult child contact among black elderly parents. *The Gerontologist* **32**(2), 213–18.

Standing, G. 1986. La flexibilité du travail et la marginalisation des travailleurs agés: pour une nouvelle stratégie, *International Labour Review* **125**(3), 239–48.

Statistics Canada 1987. *Census Canada 1986: Families Part I*. Ottawa: Statistics Canada.

Stevenson, O. 1980. A special relationship? *New Age* (summer), 18–22.

Strathern, M. 1992. *After nature: English kinship in the late twentieth century*. Cambridge: Cambridge University Press.

Sullivan, O. 1986. Housing movements of the divorced and separated. *Housing studies* **1**(1), 35–48.

Taylor, F. W. 1947. *Scientific management*. New York: Harper.

Taylor, P. & A. Walker 1991. *Too old at 50*. London: Campaign for Work.

Taylor, P. & A. Walker 1993. Employers and older workers. *Employment Gazette* **101**, 371–8.

Taylor, P. & A. Walker 1994. The ageing workforce: employers' attitudes towards older workers. *Work, Employment and Society* **8**(4), 569–91.

Taylor-Gooby, P. 1987. Citizenship and welfare. In *British social attitudes: the 1987 report*, R. Jowell, S. Witherspoon, L. Brook (eds). Aldershot: Gower.

Taylor-Gooby, P. 1991. Attachment to the welfare state. In *British social attitudes: the eighth report*, R. Jowell, L. Brook, B. Taylor (eds), 23–42. Aldershot: Dartmouth Publishing.

Temkin, L. S. 1992. Intergenerational inequality. See Laslett & Fishkin (1992a), 169–205.

Thatcher, M. 1981. Speech to the WRVS National Conference *Facing the New Challenge*, 19 January, London.

The Economist 1988. Growing rich again, 19 April.

Therborn, G. & J. Roebroek 1986. The irreversible welfare state: its recent maturation, its encounter with the economic crisis, and its future prospects. *International Journal of Health Services* 16(3), 319–38.

Thirsk, J. 1976. The European debate on customs of inheritance. In *Family and inheritance: rural society in Western Europe 1200–1800*, J. Goody, J. Thirsk, E. P. Thompson (eds), 64–86. Cambridge: Cambridge University Press.

Thomas, K. 1976. Age and authority in early modern England. *Proceedings of the British Academy* LXII, 205–48.

Thompson, L., K. Clark, W. Gunn 1985. Developmental stage and perceptions of intergenerational continuity. *Journal of Marriage and the Family* 47, 913–20.

Thomson, D. 1989. The welfare state and generation conflict: winners and losers. See Johnson et al. (1989), 33–56.

Thomson, D. 1991. *Selfish generations? The ageing of New Zealand's welfare state.* Wellington, NZ: Bridget Williams.

Thomson, D. 1992. Generations, justice, and the future of collective action. See Laslett & Fishkin (1992a), 206–35.

Timaeus, I. 1986. Family and households of the elderly population: prospects for those approaching old age. *Ageing and Society* 6(3): 271–94.

Tough, A. 1983. Self-planned learning and major personal change. In *Adult learning and education*, M. Tight (ed.), 145–52. Beckenham: Croom Helm.

Townsend, P. 1979. *Poverty in the United Kingdom*. Harmondsworth: Penguin.

Treas, J. & V. Bengston 1987. The family in later years. In *Handbook of marriage and the family*, M. B. Sussman & S. K. Steinmetz (eds), 625–48. New York: Plenum Press.

Trinder, C. 1990. *Employment after 55*, Discussion Paper 166. London: National Institute for Economic and Social Research.

Trinder, C., G. Hulme, U. McCarthy 1992. *Employment: the role of work in the third age*, Report for the Carnegie Inquiry into the Third Age, London.

Troll, L. E. (ed.) 1986. *Family issues in current gerontology*. New York: Springer.

Troll, L. & D. Smith 1976. Attachment through the lifespan. *Human Development* 19, 156–70.

Troll, L. & J. Stapley 1985. Elders and the extended family system: health, family, salience and affect. In *Lifespan and change in a gerontological perspective*, J. Munnichs et al. (eds), 50–61. New York: Springer.

Twigg, J. 1989. Models of carers: how do social care agencies conceptualise their relationships with carers? *Journal of Social Policy* 18(1), 53–66.

Uhlenberg, P. & M. Myers 1986. Divorce and the elderly. See Troll (1986), 350–61.

Ungerson, C. 1987. *Policy is personal: sex, gender and informal care*. London: Tavistock.

United Nations 1956. *The ageing of populations and its economic and social implications*. New York: UN.

Van der Veen, W. J. & Van Poppel, F. 1992. Institutional care for the elderly in the 19th century: old people in The Hague and their institutions. *Ageing and Society* 12, 185–212.

Vermulst, A., A. de Brock, R. van Zutphen 1991. Transmission of parenting across the generations. In *The psychology of grandparenthood: an international perspective*, P. K. Smith (ed.), 100–22. London: Routledge.

Waerness, K. 1990. Informal and formal care in old age: what is wrong with the new ideology in Scandinavia today? In *Gender and caring: work and welfare in Britain and Scandinavia*, C. Ungerson (ed.). Hemel Hempstead: Harvester Wheatsheaf.

Walker, A. 1981. Towards a political economy of old age. *Ageing and Society* 1(1), 73–94.

Walker, A. 1982. The social consequences of early retirement. *Political Quarterly* 53(1), 61–72.

Walker, A. 1984. *Older workers and retirement in the Sheffield steel industry*, Report to the ESRC (G 01250004), January, Sheffield.

Walker, A. 1985. Early retirement: release or refuge from the labour market? *Quarterly Journal of Social Affairs* 1(3), 211–29.

Walker, A. 1986. The politics of ageing in Britain. In *Dependency and interdependency in old age: theoretical perspectives and policy alternatives*, C. Phillipson, M. Bernard, P. Strang (eds), 46–53. London: Croom Helm.

Walker, A. 1987. Enlarging the caring capacity of the community: informal support networks and the welfare state. *International Journal of Health Services* 17(3), 369–86.

Walker, A. 1990a. The economic "burden" of ageing and the prospect of intergenerational conflict. *Ageing and Society* 10(4), 377–96.

Walker, A. 1990b. Les politiques de retraites dans la communauté européenne. *Revue Française des Affaires Sociales* 44(3), 113–26.

Walker, A. 1990c. The strategy of inequality: poverty and income distribution in Britain 1979–89. In *The social effects of free market policies: an international text*, I. Taylor (ed.), 29–48. London: Harvester Wheatsheaf.

Walker, A. 1991. The relationship between the family and the state in the care of older people. *Canadian Journal on Aging* 10(2), 94–112.

Walker, A. 1992. Thatcherism and the new politics of old age. See Myles & Quadagno (1992), 19–35.

Walker, A. 1993a. Poverty and inequality in old age. In *Ageing in society*, 2nd edn, J. Bond, P. Coleman, S. Peace (eds), 280–83. London: Sage.

Walker, A. 1993b. Community care policy: from consensus to conflict. In *Community care: a reader*, J. Bornat, C. Pereira, D. Pilgrim, F. Williams (eds), 204–26. London: Macmillan in association with the Open University.

Walker, A. 1993c. *Age and attitudes*. Brussels: Commission of European Communities.

Walker, A. 1994. *The need for solidarity between the generations*. London: National Pensioners' Convention.

235

Walker, A. 1995. *Half a century of promises*. London: Counsel and Care.

Walker, A. & P. Taylor 1993. Ageism vs productive ageing: the challenge of age discrimination in the labour market. In *Achieving a productive ageing society*, S. A. Bass, F. Caro, Y-P. Chen (eds), 61–80. Westport, Conn.: Greenwood.

Walker, A., L. Thompson, C. Morgan 1987. Two generations of mothers and daughters: role position and interdependence. *Psychology of Women Quarterly* 11, 195–208.

Walker, A., A.-M. Guillemard, J. Alber 1993. *Older people in Europe, social and economic policies*. Brussels: Commission of European Communities.

Wall, R. 1984. Residential isolation of the elderly: a comparison over time. *Ageing and Society* 4(4), 483–503.

Wall, R. 1989. The living arrangements of the elderly in Europe in the 1980s. In *Becoming and being old: sociological approaches to later life*, B. Bytheway, T. Keil, P. Allatt, A. Bryman (eds), 121–42. London: Sage.

Wall, R. 1990. Inter-generational relations in the European Past. Paper presented at British Sociological Association Conference, mimeo, Manchester.

Wall, R. 1992. Relationships between the generations in British families past and present. In *Families and households: divisions and change*, C. Marsh & S. Arber (eds), 63–85. Basingstoke: Macmillan.

Wall, R. 1994. Elderly persons and members of their households in England and Wales from pre-industrial times to the present. In *Aging in the past: demography, society and old age*, D. I. Kertzer & P. Laslett (eds). Los Angeles: University of California Press.

Wallace, S., J. Williamson, R. Garson Lung, L. Powell 1991. A lamb in wolf's clothing? The reality of senior power. In *Critical perspectives on aging*, M. Minkler & C. Estes (eds), 95–116. Amityville, New York: Baywood.

Wenger, G. C. 1984. *The supportive network*. London: Allen & Unwin.

Wenger, G. C. 1989. Support networks in old age: constructing a typology. In *Growing old in the twentieth century*, M. Jefferys (ed.), 166–85. London: Routledge.

Wenger, G. C. 1990. Elderly carers: the need for appropriate intervention. *Ageing and Society* 10(2), 197–219.

Wenger, G. C. 1992. *Help in old age: facing up to change. A longitudinal network study*. Liverpool: Liverpool University Press.

Wenger, G. C. & F. St Leger 1992. Community structure and support network variations. *Ageing and Society* 12(2), 213–36.

Westergaard, J., I. Noble, A. Walker 1989. *After redundancy: the experience of economic insecurity*. Cambridge: Polity Press.

William Salt Archaeological Society 1921. *Collections for a history of Staffordshire*. Lichfield.

Wilson, M. 1992. Forgotten people. *Social Work Today* (11 June), 15–16.

World Bank 1994. *Averting the old age crisis*. Oxford: Oxford University Press.

Wrigley, E. A. & R. Schofield 1983. English population history from family reconstitution: summary results 1600–1799. *Population Studies* 37, 157–84.

Young, M. & T. Schuller 1991. *Life after work: the arrival of the ageless society*. London: HarperCollins.

Index

Administration of Estates Act 140, 141
age cohorts 6–7, 9, 10, 14–17, 23–4, 56–80, 92, 106
  conflict 34, 35
  size 61–2
  see also generations
age discrimination *see* employment
ageing workforce 160 63
ageist attitudes 22
Americans for Generational Equity 22, 57

beneficiaries *see* inheritance
benefits 57, 59, 75
  net gains 58, 65–74, 78
  net losses 58, 74, 79
burden
  of care 101
  older people as 24
  public 19, 22, 34, 206, 208
British Mass Observation Archive 8, 81–99

capital gains 137
care 1, 54, 191 *see also* community care, residential care
  by daughters 26, 31
  by female kin 12, 105, 106
  by grandchildren 113–14
  gender differences in receipt 109

gender division of labour 28
health 19, 23, 34, 210
health and social 5, 10, 22, 30, 32, 33, 34
informal 7, 29, 100–115
statutory 101–8, 110, 117–18
carers 26
  female 3, 31, 102
caring relationship 1, 5, 8, 12, 26, 204
  and the state 28 32
  gender issues 102, 106, 109–10, 112
  normative obligations 26–7, 28
  within the family 2, 5, 8, 25, 32, 35, 100–119
censuses 41, 42, 43
cohorts *see* age cohorts
community care 33, 102, 103, 117, 215
conflict
  between employment and caring 115
  between generations 1, 2, 35, 58, 87, 109, 110
  between rich and poor 58
  between sexes 1, 58
  cohort 4, 11, 14

daughters 84, 86, 88, 115
death statistics 141–2

dementia 111
demographic
  change 13–15, 18–22, 24, 45, 55,
    79–80, 90–91, 92, 101, 113–14, 116,
    118, 125–7, 160, 189, 199, 209, 215
  timebomb 163, 181
dependency 107, 112
disablement 14, 101, 103, 105, 106,
  109, 111, 114, 116, 117
divorce and remarriage 113,
  114–15, 199

economic 1, 45, 100, 118
  analysis 8
  demographic imperative 19–22
  international agencies 7
  neo-liberal 16, 72
  obligations 2
  policy 12, 35
education 7, 56, 62, 65, 68, 69–71,
  187–205
  access to 188, 194, 197, 199, 203
  adult 191, 192, 198
  continuing 198
  for older adults 187, 189, 191,
    192, 205
  gender differences in access
    197–8, 203, 205
  intergenerational contract 205
  see also spending – social, learning
elderly 37–41, 102–13, 137, 154,
  155, 156, 157
  see also older people
employment 2, 4, 13, 16, 52, 90, 94,
  113, 115–16
  age discrimination in 162, 163,
    178, 182, 184, 185, 208
  and changing life-course 7
  changing structure of 190–91
  early exit from 160, 163
  of older workers 159–85
  of women 160
  older workers' attitudes to
    younger people 164–72
  previous status 21
  psychological effect 5
  status 164
employers' attitudes to

education 189
  younger/older people 174–84
estates 138–42
  composition of 144–7
  types of 145
  value and distribution of 142–4,
    148–51
equal opportunities 185
equity see intergenerational equity
equity release schemes 138, 145,
  158
Eurobarometer survey 3

familism 32–4
family 5, 14, 40–41, 218
  and ethnic groups 85, 92, 94, 112,
    114, 116–17
  and social class 85, 94
  attachment 82, 87
  attitudes 83, 88, 92–4
  changing values 55
  contact 83–6
  culture 91–2
  expectations 83, 97
  feelings 82, 83, 86–9
  generational patterns within 6
  multi-generational 113
  relationships 7, 10, 41, 55, 81–99,
    121, 208
  structure 12, 43, 47, 52, 94–8
feminist 102–3
fertility, decline in 5, 14, 23, 44, 57,
  209, 217
financial
  assistance 104, 109
    to children 127–33
  responsibility for aged parents 4
  support by relatives 8, 37, 45, 55
  see also transfers
friends and neighbours 102–3, 105,
  111, 116

gender see care, caring relationship,
  education
generational
  imbalances 57
  politics 218–20
  relations 8

see also intergenerational
generations   6, 7, 211–15
   contract between   1–2, 5, 61, 213
   definition of   212
   relations between   1–2, 7, 210–15
   see also age cohorts, conflict,
      welfare
grandchildren *see* care, inheritance
grandparents   89–92, 189, 199–203

health spending   70, 71, 76–8
   see also spending – social
home ownership   120–21, 124, 142,
   147, 151, 153–4, 156–8
household
   joint   106–7, 111, 118
   patterns   40, 41, 43, 47, 52, 54, 95,
      98, 105, 114
housing
   in estates   148–50
   inheritance by social class   151
   owner occupation   120
   see also equity release schemes

income support   162
informal
   caring   12, 100–19
   learning   194, 199 205
   support   100–19
   see also care
inheritance   2, 8, 113
   beneficiaries   122 32, 142, 144,
      151–2, 158
   by grandchildren   126–32
   see also estates
Inland Revenue data   8, 138–58
intergenerational
   conflict   8, 9, 22, 58, 206, 210–15
   contact   85, 216–18
   continuity   81–3
   educational contract   205
   equity   2, 11, 14, 15, 17–18, 21,
      22–5, 34, 59–65, 69, 79, 207, 210
   generativity   81–2, 98
   inequity   58–9
   relations   1–2, 7, 9, 81–99, 159,
      181, 188–9, 190–91, 194, 199
      and welfare   6, 7

and provision of care   25–34
   hostility in   185
   solidarity   33, 35, 158, 161–2,
      81–3, 89, 159
International Monetary Fund   15

Job Release Scheme   160, 171
Job Start Allowance Scheme   163

kin   3, 8, 37, 94–8
   bequests   to 122
   care by   102–119
   female   12, 28, 35, 84–5

labour force
   departure from   190
   exclusion from   162
   participation   160–61
labour market   5, 7, 14, 61
late sixties as a turning point
   47–52
learning
   economic and social context
      189–93, 198
   in work   187, 189
   life-long   187
   social roles   189, 199–203
Lichfield   41, 43, 46, 53
life chances   121, 123, 126
life course   216–19
life cycle   8, 39, 40, 65, 108, 115, 193,
   320
life expectancy   5, 10, 14, 45, 71,
   126–7, 160, 199
living arrangements
   changes in persons 65+   40–51
long-term geriatric care   12

mortality patterns   63–4, 141, 217

National Health Service   12, 35, 63
national insurance   17, 25, 56, 58,
   60, 70
new technology   165, 174, 180,
   184–5

old age   2, 38–40
   alternative transition points into
      52–3

older people   2, 14, 16–19, 23, 30
  see also burden, elderly, population
  ageing
One Child Programme in China
  108

Pay As You Go   56–8
pensions   3, 5, 15, 17, 18, 23, 34, 38,
  52, 63, 77, 204
  contract   21, 33
  contributions   5
  public   5, 10, 11, 13, 14, 15, 17, 18,
    20, 21, 34, 62, 214
  see also State Earnings Related
    Pension Scheme
  private   18, 20, 21, 56, 77
  schemes   14
  spending   23
Pensions Bill 1995   17
pensioners
  movements   21
  two generations of   33
Poor Law   5, 29, 30, 52
population
  ageing   5, 7, 9, 10, 12, 15, 20, 24,
    34, 100, 113, 206–10, 217, 219–20
  predictions $80n$
  pre-industrial   38, 40, 43, 44, 46,
    47, 53, 54
  rural   38, 41, 44, 46
poverty   14, 16, 17, 214
primogeniture   123, 124, 132

Reagonomics   16
receipts   68, 71, 75, 77–8
  and payments projection   69–78
recession   160, 183
reciprocity   2, 89, 107, 108, 111, 112,
  204
  and affect   25–8
  and affection   3, 12
recruitment   168, 178, 180–81, 185
redundancy   163, 166, 168, 182, 185
Redundancy Payment Act   162
residence patterns   47–51, 54
residential care   118, 138, 154, 193,
  215
  private   155–6

retirement   13–15, 52, 113, 126, 209
  attitude of employers to   185
  attitude of older workers to
    169–72
  early   162, 166, 168, 169, 182, 208
  flexibility   163, 173, 180, 183, 184
  of women   171, 184
  partial   173–4, 184
Rogernomics   16

siblings   83, 89, 99
social
  assistance payments   17
  contract   2–3, 5, 7, 8, 10, 11, 12,
    13–15, 33, 34
  integration   7, 35
  policy   2, 8, 12, 32, 35, 57, 101
  security   3, 13, 16, 17, 22, 23, 32,
    56, 68–71, 76, 215
  services   30, 118
  see also spending
  support   8, 37, 45, 55
Sheffield   104, 110, 115, 164
solidarity *see* intergenerational
sons   86, 88, 115
spending
  social   20, 34, 56, 59, 64–5, 69, 70,
    76, 78, 215
    patterns of   70–72
state   2, 3, 13, 218
  and intergenerational care   28–32
  ideology   8
  intervention   12
  sharing care   25
  spending   18, 101
State Earnings Related Pension
  Scheme   17, 21, 69–70
statutory care   101–8, 110, 117–18
  see also residential care
step-relationships   115

tax   2, 3, 4, 5, 13, 56, 58, 60, 65, 68,
  70, 74–7, 101, 215
  inheritance   139, 153
Thatcher government   16, 121
Thatcherism   16
third age   188–93, 204–5
trade unions   182, 185

training   188–9, 190–97
  younger workers   169
transfers   2, 12, 32, 57, 58, 59, 104, 142
  of assets   156, 158
  of resources   2, 13, 142, 208, 210
  public   13
  see also financial

unemployment   104, 115–16, 160–61, 172, 183–4, 195

voluntary work   189, 192, 203–4

voting patterns of older people   214
wealth   120–25
welfare
  and intergenerational relations   6, 8
  regimes   4
  restructuring   32–4, 35
welfare generation   8, 215
welfare state   2, 7, 8, 13–25, 56, 58–9, 63, 74, 78–80
wills   121–6
workhouse   53
Youth Training Scheme   167